TEA CLEANSE DIET

My Favorite Detox Teas to Boost Your Metabolism

(A Tasty and Easy Method for Healthy Weight Loss)

Christina Colon

Published by Sharon Lohan

Tea Cleanse Diet: My Favorite Detox Teas to Boost Your Metabolism (A Tasty and Easy Method for Healthy Weight Loss)

ISBN 978-1-990334-36-8

Legal & Disclaimer

The information contained in this book is not designed to replace or take the place of any form of medicine or professional medical advice. The information in this book has been provided for educational and entertainment purposes only.

Table of contents

Part 1

Introduction

Before investing in a 200$ tea set, or booking a flight to China to experience an authentic tea house, here's some basic tea history and knowledge to get your feet wet:

Tea is made when the leaves of the plant Camella sinensis are boiled in water. Basically, the leaves are boiled with water in a tea infuser (fancy word for teapot), and removed again in several minutes.

Camella sinensis plant takes a while to grow; it takes around three years before a new tea plant to be ready for harvesting. This isn't like growing tomatoes! When harvesting, only the top 1-2 inches of the plant are cut and used for tea. The harvested leaves and seed are known as flushes. The tea is then processed. Exactly how the tea gets processed depends what type of tea you desire (shown below).

In general, tea quality depends on two factors. The first is the height at which the plant is grown. The Traditional Chinese Tea Cultivation and Studies group concluded that tea plants grown at an altitude of around 1,500 meters, or 4,900 feet, tend to produce a better flavor. The second factor is the size of the tea leaves themselves. The smaller a tea leaf, the higher the quality (and cost) of the tea. Less really is more!

The earliest mention of tea in the Orient dates back to an ancient Chinese myth in 2737 b.c. The Chinese Emperor Shennog was boiling a large pot of water (who knows why) when tea leaves blew into the pot. After tasting this concoction (ol' Shennog was an adventurous one), he immediately fell in love with his discovery. He claimed the beverage was invigorating and promoted a sense of well-being. The popularity of tea steadily during the Han Dynasty (206b.c. - 220a.d.) in China, and by the 8th century the Chinese writer Lu Yu created the first book on the subject of tea. It was called the Ch'a Ching, translated as 'Tea Classic'.

Around this time, tea was introduced to Japan though Buddhist monks who came to China to study. These monks brought tea leaves back to their home island, where demand for tea rose faster than a Chinese firework! From there, tea was introduced to India, Britan, and other parts of the world. However, it is in the Orient that tea has its true roots.

The Many Different Types Of Tea

Green Tea

This kind of tea is extremely popular and it contains catechins, which is an antioxidant.

A lot of people drink green tea because of the potential benefits, which includes playing a role in decreasing your risk of getting cardiovascular disease.

It is also worth pointing out that some people drink green tea because they believe that you can lose weight by drinking green tea.

One of the reasons why green tea is thought to help people lose weight is because it boosts the metabolic rate.

Black

Black is one of the most commonly drank teas, and it does contain quite a bit of caffeine, at least when compare to other types of tea.

There are two antioxidants that are found in black tea, and these two have been known to lower cholesterol levels.

Also, if you drink three or more cups of this kind of tea on a daily basis, then you could end up cutting your risk of stroke by up to 21 percent.

White

If you are looking for a really healthy tea, then look no further than white tea. White tea contains catechins, just like green tea. Consuming white tea on a regular basis may even reduce the risk of having a recurrence of cancer in breast cancer survivors.

Asides from that, this kind is the purest of all teas, and it is the least processed of them all.

White tea is not fermented, and the leaves that are used to make it are dried naturally, usually via sun drying or steaming methods.

Don't worry about whether or not this tea has a plain taste to it because it does have a slight sweetness to it, so you will love drinking it.

Oolong

This tea is often served in Chinese restaurants, and it is known being very flavorful, so if you want to drink a tea with a sweet taste to it, then Oolong tea is for you.

You should know that Oolong tea is expensive, and most Oolongs come from Taiwan and it is only semi-fermented. Many drinkers prefer to drink it without milk, lemon or sugar.

This isn't because they don't like sugar, lemon or milk, it is because this kind of tea has a very delicate flavor.

Pu Erh

Pu Erh has a very rich and smooth taste to it, and the aging process lasts for a longtime. Sometimes the process can take years to complete, or it can take as little as a few months.

As for what the health benefits are, there are a number of them, and this includes playing a role in lowering your cholesterol levels, as well as help your digestion.

One of the things that make this tea stand out from other teas is that it is fermented twice, and then it is matured.

A lot of people do drink Pu Erh Tea for pleasure, but there are also many people who drink it for medicinal purposes.

Flavored

People brew tea from various things, including berries, onions, peach leaves and orange peels. Certain types of flowers are also used for tea. Herbs, spices and oils are often used too.

If you are looking for teas that have unique tastes to it, or you just want tea with some strong flavor to it, then you will want to get your hands on some flavored tea.

Blends

Blends are teas that are not from a single lineage, hence the name. Teas that fall under this category of tea has been made with other different types of teas.

Each tea comes with their own benefits; although most of their benefits may be similar. For the most part, depending on what type of tea it is, it can improve brain functions, decrease the chance of cancer, cardiovascular diseases and diabetes, relief stress, strengthen bones, aid weight loss, improve skin, aid digestion, relief cramps and spasms, and act as a sleep aid. That means, drinking tea can make one smarter in some ways. Drinking tea is beneficial for many organs, especially the heart. It can help others relax, not stress, and not go through depression. Less caffeine in tea means less sugar and a lesser change to get type 2 diabetes.

For best results, each type of tea should be prepared differently as well. The basic types of tea are:

White: Is wilted, and unoxidized.

Boiled at 65 to 70 °C (149 to 158 °F) for 1-2 minutes.

Yellow: Is unwilted and unoxidized, and left to turn a yellow color.

Boiled at 70 to 75 °C (158 to 167 °F) for 1-2 minutes.

Green: Is unwilted and unoxidized.

Boiled at 75 to 80 °C (167 to 176 °F) for 1-2 minutes.

Oolong: Is wilted and brusied; partially oxidized.

Boiled at 80 to 85 °C (176 to 185 °F) for 2-3 minutes.

Black: Is wilted, often crushed, and completely oxidized.

Boiled at 99 °C(210 °F) for 2-3 minutes.

Herbal:

Boiled at 99 °C(210 °F) for 3-6 minutes.

Chapter 1: Loss Weight With Tea

Proper diet and exercise and even counting calories are still the long-standing approaches to weight loss problems. But the issue seems to have reached a point where pharmaceutical products had to be developed to directly treat abnormal weight gain. Some of the more popular diet pills available today are designed to either make you less able to digest fat content in food or suppress your appetite. Fortunately there's a natural alternative to taking a pill or two. You can build the habit of drinking a cup of tea two to three times a day. Tea works better than diet pills because it simultaneously provides the anti-obesity mechanisms that such pills singularly offer. So with every cup you're already enabling your body to deal with fats and curb your appetite. That's just for weight control, one set of benefits among a host of others that green tea delivers.

Lessen fat digestion

There's nothing wrong with fats per se. This macronutrient along with carbohydrates is after all one of the fuel sources that your body breaks down and processes to produce energy. It's when too much is consumed, stored and left unused that abnormal weight gain and the problems that come with it happen. Lipases are the type of enzymes that, among other functions, play a role in metabolizing fats. Gastric and pancreatic lipases are the ones that directly perform this operation. These are also the lipases that the catechins in green tea inhibit. One in vitro study was able to show how a green tree extract containing 25% of the catechins was able to reduce the gastric lipase breakdown of fats by around 96% and partially do the same for pancreatic lipase at 66%. Why is this important for someone trying to control his or her weight? When fats in food aren't properly broken down in the digestive system, they can't get absorbed and just pass through. That means less additional burden to what may already be abundant stores of fat tissue.

Follow up research on the study mentioned was done, this time with human participants. The subjects were described as moderately obese. After three months of taking the same green tea extract, they experienced a 4.6 % reduction in body weight and their waists were smaller by 4.48 %. In the in vitro study mentioned earlier, it only took 60 mg of the green tea extract formulated with 25% catechins to produce the significant gastric fat breakdown reduction. Imagine what weight loss effects can be achieved by ingesting more concentrated forms. Eating as well as drinking green tea can actually provide more of these beneficial substances.

Curb appetite

The feeling of satiety is brought about by a complex process that involves the interaction of hormones, peptides, and other chemicals that send and receive nerve signals. As it turns out, the substances in green tea seem to be able to affect this process. Researchers on a study that was investigating the impact of green tea on glucose, insulin and satiety levels were somewhat surprised that the participants who took in green tea along with a meal felt fuller and had no desire to eat more.

After eliminating other possible causes, they theorized that the green tea catechins enabled the neurotransmitter called norepinephrine to act longer on the brain and establish the feeling of satiety. The reason is that the catechins blocked the enzyme (catechol-o-methyl-transferase) that breaks down the neurotransmitter. Lessening the digestion of fat and suppressing appetite is actually just two of the weight loss benefits that green tea can offer.

USE GREEN TEA TO INCREASE EXERCISE ENDURANCE

Exercise is a way of life for many people, but so is tiring quickly. In order to keep fit and healthy it's essential that regular exercise is undertaken, but to prevent the dreaded burn out there's a surprising little helper – green tea. Among the many other benefits of green tea, it can be used to: increase exercise endurance, improve performance, and prolong workout sessions. Studies are confirming this fact as well, with one having been conducted by Murase et al. The researchers wanted to look at the effects of green tea catechins in relation to endurance, fat oxidization and energy metabolism, using mice as subjects. Over a 10-week period the mice were given different levels of green tea extract and then had to swim to exhaustion, with results showing that the mice that were fed higher doses of green tea could swim for 8-24% longer. This shows the increased endurance effects of green tea, with researchers also finding that higher doses led to reduced respiratory quotients and increased levels of fat oxidization. So, as well as being a great way to increase exercise endurance, the results also indicate that green tea can be good for overall fitness and fat loss. But why is that? A lot of people think it's the caffeine content that keeps us going, and while that could quite possibly play a part it seems that there's a bit more to it than that. As with a lot of the benefits of green tea, it largely comes down to the antioxidants contained within it. The above study even focused part of its research on the effects of epigallocatechin gallate, a primary antioxidant of green, finding that the endurance-enhancing effects of green tea were largely down to this one catechin. Don't be put off by the fact that the study was conducted on mice. Murase estimates that for an athlete to see the same effects as was apparent in the study, they'd have to drink just four cups of green tea a day. And, it's also worth noting that a single high dose of green tea catechins won't do the trick. The study showed that this didn't affect performance at all. Rather, it's the long-term consumption of green tea that will have the most effect. As it only requires four cups a day, it's hardly a major lifestyle inconvenience.

So, green tea really can be used to increase exercise endurance. It would be a great dietary addition for athletes who want to improve their performance, or even for novices who want to get started with a bit of a helping hand. Either way, green tea is incredibly beneficial. As it has plenty of other health benefits, it's a great addition to anyone's diet with numerous studies confirming it.

THE EFFECTS OF GREEN TEA ON WEIGHT LOSS

Green tea has long been thought to have a number of health benefits, and the fact that it can even be used as a way to help weight loss has many dieters clamoring to get their hands on it. But can green tea live up to its claims of being a useful weight loss aide? That's what scientists are trying to find out. So far, studies into the effects that green tea can have on weight loss seem to be promising. There are a lot of studies indicating that just adding green tea into our diet can have a significant impact on our ability to lose weight, with one being published in the American Journal of Clinical Nutrition in 2005. In the study, conducted in Tokyo by Nagao et al, participants were given 690 mg catechins (a type of antioxidant found in green tea) per day. After 12 weeks participants displayed significantly reduced levels of body fat, with researchers concluding that daily consumption of green tea could therefore be beneficial in the fight to lose weight and in the prevention of obesity.

Other studies offer similar findings. One study, which was conducted in Japan by Shimotoyodome et al in 2005, used mice as test subjects and divided them into five groups. Each were fed a high-fat diet with one group receiving daily green tea extract, another one green tea extract plus exercise, and the rest being given varying levels of exercise but no green tea. The results were quite astounding despite the high-fat diet, the mice that had the green tea extract exhibited a 47% reduction in weight gain and those who had the extract plus exercise showed a massive 89% reduction. Although this study was conducted with mice, it wouldn't be so hard to envisage the same type of effects being possible with humans, as shown in other studies. This indicates that just drinking green tea can help to prevent us from gaining weight even if we don't alter our diet in any other way. Of course eating a healthy diet as well would be even more beneficial! So, what could be causing these weight loss effects? A number of theories are being offered, with just one of them being the ability of green tea to raise our metabolism. Green tea contains caffeine, and drinking moderate amounts of caffeine can increase our metabolism and thus our ability to burn more fat. The caffeine content also means that we'll be more energetic, which, subsequently, can lead to increased levels of activity and as such increased levels of calorie burning.

But is it just the level of caffeine in green tea that means we burn more energy? Actually, there's more to it than that. In a study conducted by the Department of Physiology at the University of Geneva in 1999, participants were randomly given green tea extract plus caffeine, just caffeine or a placebo on different days. The results showed that the participants expended more energy and burned far more calories on the days that they were given green tea plus caffeine than they did on any other days, indicating that there are other factors in green tea besides its caffeine content that give rise to its ability to help us lose weight and expend energy. It could be down to antioxidants instead. The antioxidants contained in green tea, particularly catechins, raise our metabolism by encouraging a process known as thermogenesis – the raising of our body temperature leading to an increase in the number of calories being burned – meaning that this could also have an impact in the ability of green tea to reduce weight. So, green tea really can be beneficial in our attempts to lose weight. Researchers suggest that drinking around 5-6 cups of green tea per day can have the most benefit, and if you substitute your regular tea or coffee for green tea then you're sure to notice the effects. Make sure to give green tea a go and see if it can help you in your weight loss quest.

Chapter 2: Health Benefits Of Tea

Put down those saucer cups and get chugging — tea is officially awesome for your health. But before loading up on Red Zinger, make sure that your "tea" is actually tea. Real tea is derived from a particular plant (Camellia sinensis) and includes only four varieties: green, black, white, and oolong. Anything else (like herbal "tea") is an infusion of a different plant and isn't technically tea.

But what real tea lacks in variety, it makes up for with some serious health benefits. Researchers attribute tea's health properties to polyphenols (a type of antioxidant) and phytochemicals. Though most studies have focused on the better-known green and black teas, white and oolong also bring benefits to the table. Read on to find out why coffee's little cousin rocks your health.

Tea has been an important beverage for thousands of years and has been a huge part of culture in countries around the world, forming major parts of ceremonies, trade routes and even starting revolutions. But tea isn't just appreciated for its good taste and worldwide appeal, it also offers numerous health benefits. Here are a few health conscious reasons you should add a cup of tea to your daily routine.

Overall Health

Tea can be beneficial to your whole body as you can see from these great effects.

Tea contains antioxidants. Antioxidants can help slow down aging and help your cells to regenerate and repair. Teas of all varieties contain high levels of antioxidant polyphenols that can help keep your body healthier and some studies suggest even ward of some cancers.

Tea has less caffeine than coffee. While there are some potential health benefits to consuming moderate amounts of caffeine, drinking loads of it is hard on your heart and other organs. Tea can provide the pick me up of coffee but without the high levels of caffeine making you less jittery and helping you get to sleep when you want.

Tea helps keep you hydrated. Conventional wisdom held that caffeinated beverages actually dehydrated you more than they hydrated you. Recent research has shown, however, that caffeine doesn't make a difference unless you consume more than 5 to 6 cups at a time. Tea has been shown to actually be more healthy for you than water alone in some cases because it hydrates while providing antioxidants.

Mental Health

Boost your brain and mental state with these benefits of tea.

Tea can create a calmer but more alert state of mind. Studies have shown that the amino acid L-theanine found in the tea plant alters the attention networks in the brain and can have demonstrable effects on the brain waves. More simply, tea can help you relax and concentrate more fully on tasks.

Tea lowers the chance of having cognitive impairment. Research on Japanese adults who consumed at least 2 cups of green tea daily found that those individuals had cut their risk of cognitive impairment by half.

Tea lowers stress hormone levels. Black tea has been shown to reduce the effects of a stressful event. Participants in a study experienced a 20% drop in cortisol, a stress hormone, after drinking 4 cups of tea daily for one month.

Tea eases irritability, headaches, nervous tension and insomnia. Red tea, also known as rooibos, is an herbal tea that originated in Africa. It has been show to have many relaxing effects that help reduce a wide range of irritations and inflammations on the body.

Tea can cause a temporary increase in short term memory. Not feeling on your game today? Try drinking some tea. The caffeine it contains may give you the boost you need to improve your memory, at least for a few hours.

Heart and Other Organs

Help protect your heart and other organs with these beneficial effects of tea.

Tea may reduce your risk of heart attack and stroke. Tea helps to prevent the formation of dangerous blood clots which are very often the cause of heart attacks and strokes. Some studies have even found that black tea drinkers were at a 70 percent lower risk of having a fatal heart attack.

Tea protects your bones. You don't have to put milk in your tea for it to help out your bones. Studies have shown that regular tea drinkers have stronger bones than those of non tea drinkers, even when other variables were adjusted for. Scientists have theorized it may be a benefit of the phytochemicals in tea.

Tea may protect against heart disease. While more studies are needed for conclusive evidence, it has been suggested that regular consumption of green and black tea leads to a significant reduction in the risk of heart disease related heart attacks.

Tea can help lower cholesterol.A recent study in China has shown that the combination of a low-fat diet and tea produced on average a 16% drop in bad cholesterol over 12 weeks when compared to a control group simply on a low-fat diet. If you're struggling to get your cholesterol under control, try adding tea to your diet to see if it helps.

Tea can help lower blood pressure. Drinking only half a cup of green or oolong tea a day could reduce your risk of high blood pressure by up to 50% and those that drink more can even further reduce their risk, even if they have additional risk factors.

Tea aids in digestion. Tea has been used in China for thousands of years as an after-meal digestive aid and it can help you as well due to the high levels of tannins it contains.

Tea helps inhibit intestinal inflammation. The polyphenols in green tea have been shown to have an effect on the intestinal inflammation caused by conditions like Irritable Bowel Syndrome allowing sufferers more comfort from a natural remedy.

Tea can reduce stomach cramps. Properties of red tea cause it to acts as anti-spasmodic agent and allowing it to aid in the relief of stomach cramps or even colic in infants.

Fitness and Appearance

Tea can not only help you feel good but look good too.

Tea helps protect your smile. While the stereotype of the tea-drinking Brits with horrible teeth may make you think otherwise, tea actually contains fluoride and tannins, both of which help reduce plaque buildup and tooth decay. Combined with a good dental hygiene regimen, this could keep your teeth healthier for longer.

Tea is calorie-free. Tea itself has no calories unless you choose to add sweeteners or milk, making it a satisfying, low-cal way to wake up and maybe even shed a few pounds.

Tea increases your metabolism. Is a slow metabolic rate keeping you from losing the weight you want? Some studies suggest that green tea may be able to boost your metabolic rate slightly, allowing you to burn an additional 70-80 calories a day. While this may not seem like much, over time it could add up.

Tea helps keep your skin acne-free. The antioxidants in green tea may have an effect on acne, and in some cases have been shown to work as well as a 4% solution of the much more harsh benzoyl peroxide.

Tea can help bad breath. A study at the University of Chicago has suggested that the polyphenols in tea can help to keep the bacteria that causes bad breath in check.

Illness and Disease

Check out these benefits of tea which may help prevent you from getting sick.

Tea strengthens your immune defenses. You may want to drink a cup of tea the next time a cold is going around your office. A recent study compared the immune activity in coffee drinkers to that of tea drinkers and found it to be much higher (up to five times) in those that chose tea. While it's no guarantee against a cold, it sure couldn't hurt.

Tea protects against cancer. While the exact types of cancer tea protects against are debated, recent research has suggested that lung, prostate and breast cancer see the biggest drop when green tea is consumed regularly. Again, there is no surefire way to prevent getting cancer, but having a cup of tea a day may is definitely worth the preventative benefits.

Tea can help prevent arthritis. Research suggests that older women who are tea drinkers are 60 percent less likely to develop rheumatoid arthritis than those who do not drink tea. The same effect has not been measured in older males, however, but additional studies may prove otherwise.

Tea can help fight the flu. Black tea may bolster your efforts to fight the flu as participants in a study who gargled with a black tea extract solution twice daily where more immune to the flu virus than those who didn't.

Tea helps fight infection. Tea contains chemicals called alkylamine antigens which act similarly to some tumor cells and bacteria, boosting the body's immune response. It has even been shown to have an effect on severe infections like sepsis.

Tea may reduce the risk of Parkinson's Disease. New studies are suggesting that regular tea consumption may help protect the body from developing this neurological disorder.

Tea can prevent food poisoning. Catechin, one of the bitter ingredients found in green tea has been shown to effectively kill the bacteria which cause food poisoning and minimize the effects of the toxins that are produced by those bacteria.

Tea can lead to the inhibition of HIV. New research from the Journal of Allergy and Clinical Immunology has found that a substance found in green tea may inhibit the HIV virus from binding and can be a healthy part of a suppression regiment.

Tea may help prevent diabetes. There is some evidence to suggest that green tea helps lower the risk of getting Type 2 Diabetes, though future research is needed to confirm the association.

Tea can lower blood sugar. Tea contains catechin and polysaccharides which have been demonstrated to have a noticeable effect on lowering blood sugar.

Tea can prevent iron damage. Those suffering from iron disorders like haemochromatosis may be helped by drinking tea, which contains tannins that limit the amount of iron the body can absorb.

Tea can help with nasal decongestion. If you've got a bit of a cold, drinking black tea with lemon may help clear up some of the congestion that's bothering you.

Just make sure your body doesn't become dependent on the treatment.

More Great Health Benefits of Tea

Anti-Cancer - Multiple studies have shown that the antioxidant compounds in tea have cancer fighting characteristics. Tea also provides inhibitory effects on DNA synthesis of leukemia cells and lung carcinoma cells. Tea has been linked to being both preventative and combative against many different types of cancer.

Anti-Heart Disease - Green tea has been shown to fight obesity and lower LDL "bad" cholesterol-two risk factors for heart disease and diabetes. Tea has also been shown to improve blood vessel function.

Anti-Stroke - Research presented at the International Stroke Conference in February 2009 found that drinking three or more cups of tea per day can reduce the risk of suffering a stroke by as much as 21%. The research, conducted at the University of California, Los Angeles, found that drinking green and black varieties of teas has a significant impact on the risk of stroke and cardiovascular disease.

Anti-Arthritis - Tea has been shown to provide rheumatoid arthritis prevention and relief.

Increased Mental Awareness - The amino acid L-theanine, which is found almost exclusively in the tea plant, affects the brain's neurotransmitters and increases alpha brain-wave activity. The result is a calmer, yet more alert, state of mind.

Weight Loss - In clinical trials conducted by the University of Geneva and the University of Birmingham it was found that tea raises metabolic rates, speeds up fat oxidation and improves insulin sensitivity. In addition, green tea contains catechin polyphenols that raise thermogenesis (the production of heat by the body), and hence increases fat expenditure.

Immune System - L-theanine may help the body's immune system response when fighting infection, by boosting the disease-fighting capacity of gamma delta T cells.

Lowered Stress Levels - Drinking black tea can lead to lower levels of the stress hormone cortisol. Blood platelet activation, which is linked to blood clotting and the risk of heart attacks has also been shown to be lower for tea drinkers.

Oral Health- Researchers at the University of Illinois, Chicago conducted a study which revealed that polyphenols found in tea help inhibit the growth of bacteria that cause bad breath, and can inhibit the creation of dental cavities.

Cardiovascular Health- Research has shown that black tea improves blood vessel reactivity, reducing both blood pressure and arterial stiffness, indicating better overall cardiovacular health.

Tea seems to be a natural and pleasant way to increase whole body health and well being, both mentally and physically. In addition to the studies conducted revealing the great health benefits of tea...the mere act of making a cup of tea...and sitting down to enjoy it, seems to have a profound effect on body, mind, and soul. This effect maybe isn't something best measured by science. Rather, it is just something that we feel.

Chapter 3: 14 Day Tea Cleanse Plan

16 WAYS TO LOSE 15 POUNDS WITH TEA IN 14 DAYS

It describes an easy and effective protocol for stripping away belly fat fast, you don't necessarily have to follow it exactly. Here are some of the most effective hacks to use when you're ready to lose weight—at the sound of a whistle.

1 FOCUS ON GREEN TEA

Every tea has its own special weight-loss powers, but if your boat is sinking and you can only grab one package of tea before swimming to the deserted island, make it green tea. Green tea is the bandit that picks the lock on your fat cells and drains them away, even when we're not making the smartest dietary choices. Chinese researchers found that green tea significantly lowers triglyceride concentrations (potentially dangerous fat found in the blood) and belly fat in subjects who eat fatty diets. Follow these steps to Make the Perfect Cup of Green Tea!

2 MAKE IT YOUR POST-WORKOUT DRINK

Brazilian scientists found that participants who consumed three cups of the beverage every day for a week had fewer markers of the cell damage caused by resistance to exercise. That means that green tea can also help you recover faster after an intense workout. In another study—this one on people—participants who combined a daily habit of four to five cups of green tea each day with a 25-minute workout for 11 days lost an average of two more pounds than the non-tea-drinking exercisers.

3 UPGRADE TO MATCHA

The concentration of EGCG—the superpotent nutrient found in green tea—may be as much as 137 times greater in powdered matcha tea. EGCG can simultaneously boost lipolysis (the breakdown of fat) and block adipogenesis (the formation of new fat cells). One study found that men who drank green tea containing 136 milligrams of EGCG—what you'd find in a single 4-gram serving of matcha—lost twice as much weight than a placebo group and four times as much belly fat over the course of three months

4 PREGAME WITH TEA

Before you head out to dinner, pour yourself a cup of green tea. The active ingredient in green tea, EGCG, boosts levels of cholecystokinin, or CCK, a hunger-quelling hormone. In a Swedish study that looked at green tea's effect on hunger, researchers divided up participants into two groups: One group sipped water with their meal and the other group drank green tea. Not only did tea-sippers report less of a desire to eat their favorite foods (even two hours after sipping the brew), they found those foods to be less satisfying.

5 DRINK TEA RIGHT BEFORE BED

You probably already know that chamomile tea can help induce sleep (there's even a brand called Sleepy Time). But science is showing that teas actually work on a hormonal level to lower our agita and bring peace and slumber. Studies have found that herbal teas like valerian and hops contain compounds that can actually reduce levels of stress hormones in our bodies, bringing on sleep — and reducing the body's ability to store fat!

6 AND DRINK IT RIGHT WHEN YOU WAKE UP

A study in the International Journal of Molecular Science found that fasting overnight, followed by green tea intake (at least 30 minutes before your first meal of the day), allowed for the best possible absorption of EGCG, the magic nutrient in green tea.

7 DRINK RED WHEN YOU'RE SEEING RED

Red tea, also known as rooibos, is a great choice for when you're struggling with midday stress. What makes rooibos particularly good for soothing your mind is the unique flavanoid called Aspalathin. Research shows this compound can reduce stress hormones that trigger hunger and fat storage and are linked to hypertension, metabolic syndrome, cardiovascular disease, insulin resistance and type 2 diabetes.

8 MEET A FRIEND FOR TEA

A new study in the journal Hormones and Behavior found that those who feel lonely experience greater circulating levels of the appetite-stimulating hormone ghrelin after they eat, causing them to feel hungrier sooner. Over time, folks who are perennially lonely simply take in more calories than those with stronger social support networks.

9 KEEP IT IN THE DARK

The active ingredients in teas are highly unstable under sunlight. Keep tea in a dark, dry place. Storing tea in sealed packaging in cool, dark conditions helps increase shelf life. If you brew iced tea, it will stay good for about 4 days, as long as you keep it refrigerated.

10 MAKE A FAT-MELTING DRESSING

To add the power of green tea's catechins on top, steep tea bags in oils (or vinegars) to create richly flavored salad dressings. A study in Nutrition Journal found that those who ate monounsaturated fats at lunch reported a 40 percent decreased desire to eat for hours afterward. Check out these Delicious Recipes Using Matcha Green Tea!

11 BLEND IT INTO A SMOOTHIE

Green or white teas make great bases for smoothies. In a study presented at the North American Association of the Study of Obesity, researchers found that regularly drinking smoothies in place of meals increased a person's chances of losing weight and keeping it off longer than a year. Add your favorite tea to one of these 56 Smoothie Recipes for Weight Loss!

12 TOSS IN SOME CHIA SEEDS

These little black morsels of nutrition are packed with fiber, protein and, most important of all, omega-3 fatty acids. Pair chia seeds with green tea in a smoothie to turbocharge the tea's fat-burning powers. According to a study review in the International Journal of Molecular Science, omega-3 polyunsaturated fatty acids may enhance not only the bioavailability of EGCG, but also its effectiveness.

13 COOK YOUR OATMEAL IN IT

Why not empower rice, quinoa and even oatmeal with the belly-fat burning properties of green tea? Tie 4 green tea bags onto a wooden spoon. Fill a small pot with 2 cups water; add wooden spoon and tea bags. Bring water to a boil and remove tea bags. Add the grains to the boiling tea water and cook as directed. Try it with these delicious Quinoa Recipes for Weight Loss!

14 PEPPER UP YOUR MEALS

When you drink tea with a salad or soup, make an effort to add some black pepper to your meal. Recent studies have indicated that a compound found in black pepper, called piperine, may help improve blood levels of EGCG by allowing it to linger in the digestive system longer — meaning that more of it is absorbed by the body.

15 MAKE A MATCHA PARFAIT

Yogurt is a great weight-loss food — until you start adding flavoring to it. Fruit-on-the-bottom teas can have as many sugar calories as a candy bar. For a fast boost of flavor, stir matcha powder into plain, full-fat Greek yogurt. Try it with one of these 25 Best Yogurts for Weight Loss!

16 TURN LEFTOVERS INTO SUPERFOODS

Ochazuke is a quickie foodie trick from Japan. It's made by pouring a cup of hot green tea over a bowl of leftover rice, then topping the bowl with savory ingredients to create a terrific slim-down lunch. Place the rice in a bowl. Pour the hot tea over it. Top with crackers, flaked salmon, seaweed, lime juice and soy sauce.

Chapter 4: 16 Delicious Tea Recipes

Smoothies

For all of these recipes, simply chuck the ingredients into your blender and give it a whiz until smooth and creamy.

Green Banana

- 1 ripe banana
- ½ cup milk
- ½ cup green tea
- 1 tbsp. agave syrup
- 1 tbsp. organic peanut butter
- 1 cup ice

Blueberry Monster

- 1 cup blueberries
- ½ cup Greek yogurt
- ½ cup green tea
- 1 tbsp. flaxseed
- 4 ice cubes

Big Orange Crush

- ¾ cup mango, frozen
- ½ cup green tea
- ½ cup carrot juice
- ½ cup Greek yogurt
- ½ cup water
- 1 tbsp. protein powder

Strawberry Papaya

- ¾ cup strawberries, frozen
- ¾ cup papaya, frozen
- ½ cup green tea
- ½ cup milk
- 1 tbsp. fresh mint leaves

Punchy Pineapple

- 1 cup pineapple, frozen
- ½ cup Greek yogurt
- ½ cup green tea
- ½ cup milk

Big Green Goddess

- ¼ pitted and peeled avocado
- 1 tbsp. organic honey
- 1 ripe banana
- ½ cup green tea
- ½ cup ice
- 1 scoop of protein powder

Optional ingredient– 1 tsp. ginger, fresh grated

Meals

Black Bean Omelet

Ingredients

- 14-16 oz. can drained black beans
- ¼ tsp. cumin
- Juice from one lime
- 8 eggs
- ½ cup + extra feta cheese
- Salt and pepper to taste
- Hot sauce to taste
- Bottled salsa

Method:

1. Put the beans, cumin, lime and a bit of hot sauce into your blender and whiz until you have something the consistency of refried beans– add water if necessary
2. Heat a little olive oil or butter in a pan

3. Beat two eggs with salt and pepper and add them to the pan
4. Stir and lift the eggs to cook thoroughly
5. Add¼ tsp. of bean mixture and 2 tbsp. feta down the center of the omelet
6. Fold one-third over and then the other third; serve hot
7. Repeat with the rest of the ingredients to make more
8. Garnish with feta and salsa

Prosciutto and Fig Salad

Ingredients:

- 12 cups baby arugula
- 8 whole figs
- 6 slices prosciutto in thin strips
- ¼ cup toasted pine nuts
- ½ cup fresh goat cheese, crumbled
- Salt and pepper to taste
- Balsamic vinaigrette

Method

1. Mix the figs, arugula, nuts and cheese in a bowl with a little salt and black pepper
2. Add enough of the vinaigrette to coat the arugula and toss before serving

Chicken with Sesame Noodles

Ingredients

- 6 oz. fettuccine, whole wheat
- 2 tsp. + extra toasted sesame oil
- 2 tbsp. warm water
- 1½ tbsp. organic peanut butter, chunky
- 1½ tbsp. soy sauce, low sodium
- 2 tsp. chili sauce
- 2 cups cooked chicken, shredded
- Juice of 1 lime
- 1 sliced bell pepper, red or yellow
- 2 cups sugar snap peas

Optional ingredients– 1 cup shelled cooked edamame

Method

1. Boil a large pan of salted water and add the fettuccine– cook as per instructions on pack
2. Drain and toss with a little sesame oil
3. Mix the water, lime juice, soy sauce, peanut butter, chili sauce and sesame oil together and microwave for about 45 seconds; stir well to combine
4. Toss the noodles in the sauce

5. Stir the chicken, pepper, edamame and pepper together and combine in the noodle before serving

Crab and Avocado Salad

Ingredients

- 8 oz. crab meat
- ½ cup cucumber peeled, seeded and chopped
- ½ cup red onion, minced
- ¼ cup fresh cilantro, chopped
- 1 red jalapeno pepper, minced
- 1 tbsp. fish or soy sauce
- 1 tbsp. sugar
- Juice of 1 lime
- Salt
- 4 Haas avocado, pitted and halved
- 1 lime, cut in quarters

Method

1. Mix the onion, cucumber, crab, fish sauce, jalapeno, cilantro, juice and sugar together stirring to combine– try not to break the crab up too much
2. Salt the avocado lightly and spoon the crab into the halves
3. Serve with lime

Chinese Chicken Salad

Ingredients

- ½ head red cabbage
- 1 head Napa cabbage
- ½ tbsp. sugar
- 2 cups chicken, cooked and shredded
- ½ cup Asian vinaigrette (bottled)
- 1 cup cilantro, fresh
- 1 cup mandarin orange
- ¼ cup toasted almonds, sliced
- Salt and pepper to taste

Method

1. Cut the cabbages lengthways and take the cores out
2. Slice thinly and toss in the sugar
3. Toss cold chicken in the vinaigrette and warm in the microwave
4. Add to the other ingredients, toss together and serve

Peaches and Grilled Pork

Ingredients

- 4 bone-in pork chops, 1" thick
- Olive oil
- Salt and pepper
- 2 peaches, pitted and halved
- 2 tbsp. toasted pine nuts
- 1 small thinly sliced red onion
- ½ cup blue cheese, crumbled
- 1 tbsp. balsamic vinegar

Method

1. Heat your grill
2. Brush olive oil over the chops and season
3. Grill for about 4 or 5 minutes on each side– it should be charred but not burnt on the outside
4. Brush oil over the peaches and grill them, cut side facing down, for about 5 minutes
5. Remove them and slice them
6. Toss the peaches with the rest of the ingredients
7. Spoon the mixture onto each chop and serve

Honey and Mustard Salmon

Ingredients

- 4 salmon fillets
- 1 tbsp. butter
- 1 tbsp. Dijon mustard
- 1 tbsp. brown sugar
- 1 tbsp. soy sauce
- 1 tbsp. organic honey
- ½ tbsp. olive oil
- Salt and pepper

Method

1. Preheat your oven to 400° F
2. Mix the sugar and butter together and microwave for about 30 seconds until melted
3. Add the soy sauce, honey and mustard, stirring well
4. Heat the oil and season the salmon
5. Place skin-side up in the pan and cook for 3 or 4 minutes until browned. Flip and cook the other side
6. Brush the glaze over the salmon and place in the oven; cook for about 5 minutes, until the fish is flaky but firm– don't let white fat appear on the surface
7. Remove from the oven, brush more glaze on and serve

Bagged Halibut

Ingredients

- 2 fillets of halibut
- 8 oz. marinated and drained artichoke hearts
- 1 cup cherry tomato
- 2 tbsp. chopped olives, Kalamata variety
- ½ fennel bulb, thinly sliced
- 1 lemon cut in half - half quartered, the other sliced thinly
- ¼ dry white wine
- Salt and pepper

Method

1. Preheat your oven to 400° F
2. Place each fish fillet on a sheet of parchment paper and top with an even layer of artichoke, olive, fennel, tomato and slices of lemon
3. Drizzle olive oil and wine over the top, season and wrap in the paper, sealing it up tight so the steam can't escape
4. Bake the fish for about 20 to 25 minutes and serve garnished with lemon

Shrimp and Mango Summer Rolls

Ingredients

- 1 tbsp. organic chunky peanut butter
- 1 tbsp. sugar
- 1 tbsp. fish or soy sauce
- 1 tbsp. + extra rice wine vinegar
- 2 oz. vermicelli
- 8 sheets rice paper
- ½ lb. medium shrimp, cooked and halved
- ½ thin sliced red bell pepper
- 1 peeled and pitted mango sliced into slim strips
- 4 green scallions, cut into slim strips
- ½ cup of fresh cilantro or fresh mint

Method

1. Mix the sugar, peanut butter, fish sauce, and vinegar together with 1 tbsp. warm water. Stir well and set aside
2. Cook the noodle, drain and toss with a little vinegar
3. Dip a rice paper into warm water for a couple of seconds, until warm and bendy. Lay it on a cutting board

4. Divide the ingredients into 8 and spread each portion over the rice paper, leaving½ inch at each end
5. Fold the rice paper ends in towards the middle and then roll it up like a burrito
6. Repeat with the rest and serve with the sauce

Beijing Wings

Ingredients

- ½ cup soy sauce, low sodium
- ¼ cup brown sugar
- 4 minced garlic cloves
- 1 tbsp. fresh grated ginger
- 2 lb. chicken wings
- 1 tbsp. Sriracha
- 2 tbsp. butter
- Juice from½ a lime

Optional– chopped scallions and sesame seeds

Method

1. Mix the soy sauce with 2 tbsp. brown sugar, the ginger and the garlic in a Ziploc bag
2. Add the wings and shake to coat thoroughly
3. Refrigerate for between 1 and 8 hours
4. Preheat your oven to 450° F
5. Line a baking sheet with foil and lightly oil it
6. Take the wings from the bag and lay them onto the foil
7. Roast for 15 minutes or until cooked through

8. Heat up the lime juice, Sriracha and butter, add the rest of the sugar and stir well to combine
9. Add the wings to the melted mixture and sauté for between 2 and 3 minutes or until the sauce is clinging to the meat
10. Serve garnished with the seeds and scallions if using

Chicken Pot Stickers

Ingredients

- 2 dozen pot stickers, frozen– vegetable, pork or chicken
- 1 tbsp. peanut or sesame oil
- 4 oz. sliced mushrooms
- 2 cups of trimmed snow or sugar snap peas
- 1 tbsp. rice wine vinegar
- 1 tbsp. soy sauce
- Sriracha to taste

Optional– sesame seeds

Method

1. Boil a large pan of water and add the pot stickers. Cook until soft but not gummy, a few minutes
2. Drain and leave to one side
3. Heat the oil and add the mushrooms, cooking until lightly browned
4. Add the pot stickers and cook until brown and crispy on the bottom
5. Add the snap peas and toss in the last minute of cooking

6. Take off the heat, add the Sriracha, soy sauce, and vinegar, stirring gently
7. Serve with the sesame seeds

Thai Chicken Curry

Ingredients

- 1 tbsp. canola or peanut oil
- 1 large sliced onion
- 2 cloves minced garlic
- 2 tbsp. fresh minced ginger
- 1 tbsp. red curry paste
- 14 oz. coconut milk
- 1 cup chicken stock
- 1 sweet potato, peeled and cubed
- 8 oz. green beans
- 1 lb. chicken breast, boneless and skinless cut into¼ inch strips
- Juice of 1 lime
- 1 tbsp. fish sauce
- Chopped fresh basil or cilantro for garnish
- Brown rice, steamed

Method

1. Heat the oil and sauté the garlic, ginger, and onions for about 5 minutes
2. Add the curry paste and cook for a few more minutes

3. Add the broth and milk, stir and bring up to a simmer
4. Add the potato, simmer for about 10 minutes, then stir the beans and chicken in
5. Cook for 5 minutes until the chicken is cooked and the vegetable are tender
6. Add the fish sauce and lime juice, stir in and serve over the rice. Garnish with the herbs

Sea Bass Packet

Ingredients

- 4 sea bass
- 8 asparagus spears trimmed and chopped
- 4 oz. mushrooms, shitake with stems removed
- 1 tbsp. grated fresh ginger
- 2 tbsp. soy sauce, low sodium
- 1 tbsp. Mirin Sake or a sweet white wine
- Salt and pepper

Method

1. Preheat your oven to 400° F
2. Lay out 4 large sheets of aluminum foil
3. Fold them into thirds and lay a fillet in the center
4. Scatter mushrooms, ginger and asparagus over the top and drizzle the wine and soy sauce over the top
5. Season, fold the foil over the fish, roll the ends to towards the middle and seal tightly
6. Place the packages on a baking tray and cook for about 15 or 20 minutes
7. Serve in the packets

Swordfish Grilled with Pesto

Ingredients

- 2 tbsp. pesto, bottled
- 4 swordfish steaks
- 1 tbsp. olive oil
- 2 cloves peeled and crushed garlic
- 2 cups cherry tomatoes
- Salt and pepper

Method

1. Smear pesto over the steaks, over them and leave to marinate for 30 minutes in the refrigerator
2. Heat up the oil and cook the garlic of a couple of minutes, or until light brown
3. Add the tomatoes, sauté until the skins have started to blister and season
4. Preheat the grill, season the fish and cook for 4 or 5 minutes under a hot grill. Flip the steaks and cook the other side
5. Reheat the tomato mix and serve over the top of the steak

Grilled Salmon and Ginger-Soy Butter

Ingredients

- 2 tbsp. softened unsalted butter
- ½ tbsp. chives, minced
- ½ tbsp. fresh grated ginger
- Juice from 1 lemon
- ½ tbsp. soy sauce, low-sodium
- 4 salmon fillets
- Salt and pepper
- 1 tbsp. olive oil

Method

1. Combine the lemon juice, butter, ginger, chives, and soy sauce together; set to one side
2. Preheat the grill and season the salmon, rubbing oil in as well
3. Oil the grill grates and cook the salmon, skin side down, until the skin is crisp, about 4 or 5 minutes
4. Turn and cook the other side to your taste
5. Serve with a dollop of the butter mix, allowing it to melt over the fish

Spicy Thai Chicken and Basil

Ingredients

- 1 tbsp. canola or peanut oil
- 1 thin sliced red onion
- 2 thin sliced jalapeno peppers
- 4 minced cloves of garlic
- 1 lb. chicken breast, skinless and boneless, chopped into small bits
- 1 tbsp. sugar
- 1 tbsp. soy sauce, low sodium
- 2 cups fresh basil
- Brown rice

Method

1. Heat the oil and add the jalapenos, onion and the garlic. Stir-fry for a couple of minutes, keeping it all moving
2. Add the chicken and cook until it starts to brown
3. Add the sugar, soy sauce, basil and fish sauce, stir and cook for another minute
4. Serve with brown rice

Chicken with Capers, Tomato and Olives

Ingredients

- 4 chicken breast skinless and boneless, pounded to¼ inch thickness
- Salt and pepper
- 2 cups chopped tomato
- ½ red onion, diced
- ½ cup pitted and chopped olives
- ¼ cup pine nuts
- 2 tbsp. capers
- 2 tbsp. olive oil

Optional– fresh basil, sliced thin

Method

1. Preheat your oven to 450° F
2. Season the chicken
3. Lay out four sheets aluminum foil
4. Fold each one in half and then fold up about an inch on each side to make 4 trays
5. Place a chicken breast into each tray
6. Mix the rest of the ingredients together and season
7. Spoon the mixture over the chicken

8. Bake for about 15 minutes and serve with any juices drizzled over the top and garnished with basil

Teriyaki Pork with Apple Chutney

Ingredients

- 4 pork chops
- 1 cup teriyaki marinade
- ½ tbsp. canola or peanut oil
- ½ diced onion
- 1 tbsp. fresh ginger, grated
- 1 cored and peeled apple, diced
- ¼ cup apple cider vinegar
- ½ cup apple juice
- 1 tsp. five-spice Chinese powder

Method

1. Put the marinade into a Ziploc bag
2. Add the pork chops and shake to coat
3. Marinate for between 1 and 8 hours in the refrigerator
4. Preheat the grill
5. Heat the oil over medium heat and cook the ginger and onion for a couple of minutes
6. Add the vinegar juice, apple, and Chinese powder, stir and simmer on a lower heat for 10 minutes– the apples will be soft but not mushy and the liquid should thicken a little

7. Remove the chops from the marinade, soak off the excess sauce and grill for about 5 minutes one each side until charred lightly
8. Serve with the apple chutney

Roast Pork Loin and Lemon Beans

Ingredients

- 3 cloves minced garlic
- Zest from 2 oranges
- 1 tbsp. fennel seed
- 1½ tbsp. fresh chopped rosemary
- 1 tbsp. olive oil
- 1 pork loin with a little fat on it
- Salt and pepper
- 2 16 oz. cans of white beans, drained and rinsed
- Juice from 1 lemon

Method

1. Preheat your oven to 450° F
2. Mix the fennel seed, zest, garlic and 1 tbsp. rosemary together on a chopping board. Using a knife, run it through until the mixture feels like a paste
3. Spoon it into a bowl, add the olive oil and combine
4. Season the pork and then rub the paste all over it
5. Either cook straight away or marinate for a few hours for a better flavor

6. To cook, oat for 25 or 30 minutes in a pan until you get a reading from an instant thermometer of 150° to 155° F when inserted into the middle
7. Take it out of the oven and leave to rest for 10 minutes before you slice it
8. Mix the beans with the rest of the rosemary and lemon juice and cook, warming through. Season and serve with the pork and beans

Rosemary and Garlic Roast Beef

Ingredients

- 3 lb. rump roast
- 8 peeled and halved garlic cloves
- 2 tbsp. olive oil
- ½ tbsp. fresh chopped rosemary
- Salt and pepper

Method

1. Half an hour before cooking, allow the beef to sit at room temperature
2. Reheat youroven to 250° F
3. Using a small sharp knife, make cuts into the roast, and insert garlic cloves all over it
4. Rub the olive oil over the roast and season with rosemary, salt, and pepper
5. Put onto a rack on a baking tray and cook in the center of the oven for 90 minutes
6. Turn the heat to 475° and roast for a further 15 minutes, or until the beef has turned a deep brown. A thermometer should read140° F when inserted the middle

Provençal Chicken

Ingredients

- 1 tbsp. olive oil
- 8 chicken thighs, skinless and boneless
- Salt and pepper
- 1 yellow onion, minced
- 3 minced garlic cloves
- 3 diced Roma tomatoes
- 1 cup white wine, dry
- 1 cup chicken broth
- 1 tsp. Herbs de Provence
- ¼ cup rough chopped, pitted olives, Kalamata variety
- Fresh basil for garnishing

Method

1. Heat up the oil in a sauté pan
2. Season the chicken and cook for about 6 minutes, turning once. Put to one side
3. Add the garlic, onion and tomatoes, cooking for 5 minutes or so, until the vegetables are soft
4. Add the herbs, broth and wine, bring up to a simmer and then add the chicken back in

5. Simmer for about 20 minutes, uncovered and turning the chicken once
6. Stir the olives in, garnish and serve

Herb Roasted Turkey Breast

Ingredients

- 8 cups of water
- 1 cup sugar
- ¾ cup salt
- 1 large turkey breast, skinless and boneless
- 2 clove peeled garlic
- Salt and pepper
- 1 tbsp. olive oil
- ½ tbsp. fresh rosemary, minced

Method

1. Put the sugar, salt, and water into a large pot and bring to the boil, stirring till the salt and sugar have dissolved
2. Allow to cool down to room temperatures and then add the turkey
3. Cover and leave in the refrigerator for 4 hours or more
4. Preheat youroven to 425° F
5. Take the turkey out of the liquid and pat it dry
6. Roll it up so it looks like a log and use butcher string to tie it into this shape, using three knots, each about 2 inches apart

7. Mince the garlic and mix with the oil and rosemary
8. Rub it on the turkey along with some pepper
9. Put the meat into a large pan and roast for about one hour. A thermometer inserted should read 160° F
10. Serve with traditional roast sides

STEP REFRIGERATOR TEA

- 4 tea bags
- 4 cups water

Fill a pitcher or mason jar with water. Hang tea bags in the water. Cover and steep 6-12 hours in the refrigerator. Serve as desired with any flavorings or sweeteners.

CHEAP AND EASY FLAVORED TEA RECIPE

- 3 family sized tea bags
- 4 flavored tea bags (lemon, blueberry, blackberry, mint, orange, cinnamon– Any flavor will work.)
- 1 cup sugar

Pour 4 cups boiling water over the tea bags and allow to steep for 6 minutes. Remove and squeeze the tea bags. Add sugar and stir until dissolved. Pour into a gallon pitcher and add cold water and ice to fill.

BLUEBERRY TEA RECIPE

- 1 (16-oz.) pkg. blueberries (frozen or fresh)
- 1/2 cup lemon juice
- 4 cups water
- 4 cups brewed tea
- 3/4 cup sugar

Bring the blueberries and lemon juice to a boil in a large saucepan over medium heat. Cook, stirring occasionally, for 5 minutes. Remove from the heat and pour through a fine wire-mesh strainer into a bowl, using the back of a spoon to squeeze out the juice. You can freeze the solids in ice cube trays and use for smoothies. Stir 3/4 cup sugar and the blueberry juice mixture into the tea. Pour into a pitcher. Cover and chill 1 hour. Serve over ice. Makes 4 servings.

RASPBERRY TEA RECIPE

- 1 (16-oz.) pkg. raspberries (frozen or fresh)
- 4 cups water
- 3/4 cup sugar
- 4 cups brewed tea

Bring the raspberries and water to a boil in a large saucepan over medium heat. Cook, stirring occasionally, for 5 minutes. Remove from the heat and pour through a fine wire-mesh strainer into a bowl, using the back of a spoon to squeeze out the juice. Add the tea to a pitcher. Stir in the sugar and raspberry juice mixture. Chill 1 hour. Serve over ice.

COPYCAT OLIVE GARDEN PEACH TEA RECIPE

- 1 cup sugar

- 1 cup water

- 2-3 sliced fresh peaches

- 6 cups brewed tea

Place the sugar, 1 cup of the water and the peaches into a saucepan and cook until they come to a boil. Reduce the heat to a simmer (medium). Crush the peaches as you stir to dissolve the sugar. Once the sugar is dissolved, turn off the burner, cover, and allow the mixture to rest for about 30 minutes. Strain the syrup to remove the fruit pieces. Save the fruit pieces for smoothies. Add the syrup to the tea and refrigerate. Serve over ice.

ORANGE TEA RECIPE

- 2-3 cups brewed tea, still hot
- 1 cup sugar
- 1 orange, sliced
- 1 tsp. vanilla
- Dash cinnamon

Place the oranges in the bottom of a pitcher. Add vanilla and cinnamon. Pour the tea into the pitcher while still hot so the sugar dissolves and top off with water. Serve over ice.

STRAWBERRY ICED TEA RECIPE

- 3 cups brewed tea
- 4 cups fresh or frozen strawberries
- 1 1/2 cups water
- 1 1/2 cups sugar (or sweetener of your choice)

In a saucepan, boil the strawberries, sugar, and water. Lower the heat and simmer for 10-15 minutes. Cool slightly. Pour the syrup through a fine mesh sieve into a gallon pitcher. You can freeze the solids in ice cube trays and use for smoothies.

Pour the tea into the pitcher with the syrup and stir. Fill the pitcher with cold water. Chill completely. Then serve over ice and/or freshly frozen strawberries.

EASY PEACH TEA RECIPE

- 8 cups brewed tea

- 3/4 cup sugar

- 11-ounce can peach nectar (found in the fruit juice section or alcoholic drink section)

In a 10-12 cup pitcher, pour the ingredients and stir until the sugar is dissolved. Add ice until the pitcher is full. Serve.

MINT LIME TEA COOLER

- 4 cups brewed tea
- 1 1/2 cups sugar
- Juice from 6 limes
- Fresh mint or raspberries for a flavor twist and cute garnish

Add the sugar to a one gallon pitcher. Add the brewed tea. Add enough water to equal one gallon of tea. Add the lime juice and a few mint sprigs. Stir until the sugar is dissolved. Serve over ice and garnish with mint sprigs if desired. This mint lime tea is best served cold with ice!

JOLLY RANCHER TEA RECIPE

- 1 tea bag
- 4 Jolly Ranchers, any flavor

Brew the tea and Jolly Ranchers in boiling water. Serve hot or cold over ice.

CITRUS TEA RECIPE

- 6 cups water

- 2 regular individual sized tea bags

- 6 Tbsp. honey or sugar

- 1 stick cinnamon (which gives it just the right amount of zing)

- Juice of 2 lemons

- Slices of orange, lemon, lime and/or cucumber.

Bring the water to a boil in a large saucepan, with cinnamon and sugar. Remove from the heat and drop in the tea bags. Cover and let it rest for 1 hour. Pour the tea into a pitcher, discarding the cinnamon stick. Stir in lemon juice. Add sliced fruits. Refrigerate overnight or until chilled. Add ice cubes and slices of citrus before serving.

Blackberry Tea Recipe

- 5 regular sized tea bags
- 4 cups boiling water
- 1/4 cup mint leaves, crushed
- 1/2 cup sugar
- 2 lbs. blackberries

Brew the tea and mint in boiling water. Strain. Stir in the sugar. Purée the blackberries in a blender or food processor. Strain through a fine sieve. Discard the pulp and seeds. Stir the blackberry purée into the tea.

Taste and adjust the sugar as desired. Chill. Serve over ice garnished with mint leaf and 2 or 3 blackberries.

TROPICAL ORANGE TEA RECIPE

- 6 cups refrigerator tea
- 1 2/3 cups pineapple juice
- Juice from 1 large lemon
- Juice from 1 large orange
- 1 cup sugar

Pour the tea into a pitcher. Add the pineapple juice, lemon juice, orange juice and sugar. Stir to combine. Chill the tea until you're ready to serve.

Boston Iced Tea

Ingredients:

- 2 liters water
- 1/2 cup white sugar
- 8 tea bags (black tea)
- 2 cups cranberry juice concentrate

Directions:

In a medium-sized pan or pot, bring the water to a boil. Add sugar and stir until dissolved. Remove from heat. Allow to cool for 1-2 minutes. Add teabags and steep for 5 minutes or until desired strength is achieved. Stir in cranberry juice concentrate. Allow to cool for 5-10 minutes before placing in the refrigerator. Add ice cubes before serving.

Orange Earl Grey Tea

Ingredients:

- 2 liters water
- 1/4 cup sugar
- 8 tea bags (Earl Grey Tea)
- 1 cup fresh orange juice
- 2 tablespoons sliced orange peels or peel of one orange

Directions:

In a small pan, bring 1 liter of water to a boil. Stir in sugar until fully dissolved. Remove from heat. Allow to cool for 2 minutes. Steep the teabags and orange peels for 5 minutes or until desired strength is achieved. Remove the teabags and strain the orange peels. Place on a large pitcher. Add orange juice and 1 liter of cold water. Stir. Allow cooling for 5-10 minutes before placing in the refrigerator. Add ice cubes before serving.

Honey-Lemon Iced Green Tea

Ingredients:

- 2 liters water
- 2 cups honey
- 8 teabags (green tea)
- 1 medium-sized lemon

Directions:

In a small pan or pot, bring to a boil 1 liter of water. Remove from heat and allow cooling for 3 minutes. Steep the teabags for 3 minutes or until desired strength is achieved. Remove teabags. Stir in honey. Add 1 liter of water and stir. Slice lemon into thin wedges and add to mixture. Allow to cool before placing in the refrigerator. Add ice cubes prior to serving.

Place slices of lemon or orange on the rim of the glass. Fill the glass with ice cubes before pouring the ice tea mixture.

If you are preparing this drink for a dinner party one way to really knock it out of the park, and provide the perfect chilled rink is to put the tea in the fridge to let it cool. Then about half an hour before your party begins put the pitcher in the freezer. This will bring down the core temperature and will ensure that the ice cubes don't melt right away. This avoids watering down your drink, while still having a cold beverage ready for your guests!

Chapter 5: The Do's And Don'ts On A Tea Cleanse

What is a teatox?

A teatox is a detox using tea. You detox by drinking specially formulated tea to cleanse the body.

Tea uses a blend of all-natural herbal ingredients, carefully selected, sourced, blended and expertly formulated to help maximize your body's detox ability and kick-start a healthy lifestyle.

Dos

Consult your doctor before teatoxing if you have a pre-existing medical condition

If you are under 15 years of age, you should discuss with your parents whether teatoxing is right for you

To be on the safe side, do take the pill in the morning after you have been to the toilet and had your breakfast or early in the evening, 2-3 hours before you take the Night Cleanse Tea. Please do check with your doctor if you have any doubt.

Don'ts

Teatox is not a meal-replacement program so eat regularly and don't skip meals

Do not take our tea if you are pregnant or breastfeeding as our blends are too strong for babies

Morning Boost shouldn't be drunk after 5pm as the caffeine may interfere with your sleep

Do not drink Night Cleanse tea during fasting periods as it might result in watery stools, as there is no solid food to flush out. There is also limited water intake during fasting and drinking the tea might result in further dehydration.

Chapter 6: Day 1 – Cleaning Out The Pantry

I have devoted this chapter to something really important. If you really want to lose weight and you want to do so quickly, day one should be devoted to clearing out the pantry of those things that are making you fat in the first place. This includes the following:

- Fast foods and processed foods

- Cakes, Biscuits and other temptations

- Sugar based foods

- Items that include saturated fats:

o Crisps

o Fatty meat

o Processed meats

Of course there are other foods that hamper your metabolism, but if you can avoid processed foods altogether during this week, then that's great. You may not know it but those frozen vegetables that purport to be good for your health may not be. If they have sauces or flavorings, cut those out too and stick to natural foods bought in their natural state.

During the detox, you need to avoid coffee and tea, but you can allow yourself one coffee to get yourself geared up in the morning. Make it black if at all possible and use brown sugar.

Foods you can eat

You can eat all types of healthy choices to include vegetables, fruits, lean meat, white meat and fish. Eggs are also healthy. Cheese should be eaten in moderation, since this contains saturated fats.

Try to stock up on healthy snacks and this can includes nuts and raisins, though don't overdo the nuts and avoid the salted varieties since these have been processed.

For desserts, try fresh fruit salads or even natural yogurt with a spoonful of brown sugar. Avoid white sugar. Stewed apple is rather good and you can mix this with other seasonal berries to give you a delightful taste. I actually make these myself because I prefer that they be made with fresh ingredients. If you keep your old yogurt pots and clean them out, you can make a batch at a time and keep them in the refrigerator.

Fiber

Although you may not be keen on it, fiber plays a very important part in your detox as fiber helps the food to pass through the gut sufficiently quickly so that it does not become toxic and form fat. Examples of each type of fiber are included below. One type dissolves in water and lines the stomach so that toxins cannot stick to the lining and the other does not, meaning that it pushes foods through the intestines more effectively.

Insoluble Fiber

- Whole wheat

- Couscous

- Whole grains

- Broccoli and other dark greens

- Onions

- Root vegetable skins

- Zucchini

Soluble Fiber

- Oatmeal or porridge

- Pears, Apples, Oranges, Cucumber, Celery, Carrots

- Flaxseed

- Lentils

- Oat Bran

Chapter 7: Preparing Your Tea And Understanding Its Benefits

You will need to buy Nettle Leaf Tea and this can be bought at a pharmacy, a health food store or online. The reason for suggesting this particular tea is because I have experience with using it and it has a wonderful array of good qualities that will assist you in losing weight and getting back into shape. I have outlined the good qualities of this tea in this chapter.

Preparation is simple. You need to boil two liters of water and add the leaves to it in the proportions shown on the pack. Since this is different for different makers, I cannot give exact details, but the mixture needs to be relatively weak. Simmer it for ten minutes and then take it off the heat. While this is cooling, make sure that you have a bottle suitable to contain the mixture. I use mineral water bottles, but these should be placed in the refrigerator between drinks.

Instead of drinking all of those cups of coffee and tea that you are accustomed to, replace your drinks with the tea mixture. This can be served hot or cold, though I do find that it tastes pretty neutral when it is used cold. Since you may be replacing hot drinks, you may have a preference for warmer tea and each time you want a cup, you can simply warm up sufficient for your needs.

If you do make nettle tea from the nettles in your garden, be aware to use them from areas that have not been treated with pesticides or weed killer. It is preferable in the case of fresh leaves to make sure that your leaves are adequately boiled so as to take any sting from them. With bought teas, follow the preparation instructions on the pack.

Health Benefits of Nettle Tea

Nettle tea helps you to detoxify the body because it cleans out the intestines, but it does it very gently. The reason why this affects the metabolism is because the tea makes your body more efficient at processing the foods that you consume. When the body is working as it should be, weight loss, rather than fat gain, follows. Your kidneys are able to process food easier and you will find that you feel less sluggish.

The side benefits to nettle tea are indeed diverse. It can help you to avoid cardiovascular disease by making the bodywork more efficiently. The lymphatic system gets clogged up with stored waste, as do the muscles, so drinking the tea during the course of the seven days will certainly have added benefits to the way that you feel. During the time that you drink this tea, you will find that it has diuretic values and should always make sure that you drink sufficient fresh water to compensate for that.

Although people are under the mistaken belief that losing liquids from the body is healthy, many do not drink sufficient water and this can cause dehydration. Think of it like this. An osteopath who dealt with patients on an ongoing basis informed them that if they didn't drink coffee, they would not be in the state of pain he found them in. The reason was that coffee is also a diuretic and for each cup that you drink, you can expect to lose two of three cups of liquid from the body. Diuretics keep the flow of liquid going which is good for your bladder and for your kidneys, but if you have had previous kidney function problems, it's a wise idea to consult your doctor before going on a nettle tea detox.

Other health benefits of this tea are that it helps men to avoid prostate problems and works as a protection against cancer. That's pretty powerful stuff and all this comes from nature. Phyto-therapeutic studies on the qualities of the stinging nettle are renowned worldwide, and the website **Healing Cancer Naturally** backs up my own experience by letting readers know what these values are. Used as an anti-inflammatory and known for enhancing the immune system, nettles can also help diseases such as thyroid problems, helping with bioavailable levels of testosterone as well as improving brainpower!

Thus, as well as losing weight, you will be giving your body a real chance against common ailments as well as serious illnesses by using nettle tea as your 7 day detox choice. There are so many answers that come from nature and putting your metabolism back into check will really help you to feel good and to avoid many of the pitfalls that age inflicts upon most people.

Chapter 8: Going Through The Detox

There are all kinds of arguments about when you should drink the tea to get the best benefits from it. My advice is that you drink it separately to your food. When you would normally drink tea or coffee, replace it with nettle tea. The detox process is something that should last you seven days, although you can choose to use the tea for a week every month to keep yourself in really great shape.

When you wake up in the morning, breakfast is important, but avoid eating anything that is fried. There are better alternatives. For example, try scrambled egg on whole wheat toast or cereals. The odd bowl of porridge is also a great idea because it lines the stomach and makes you ready for the day. If you do use porridge, try not to up the calorie count by adding too much maple syrup. Avoid pancakes since these are made with white flour, which will bind in your intestines, and cause blockages that you do not want during the detox period. If you like fruit juice or a smoothie, then by all means indulge, but remember that there is a lot of natural sugar in freshly squeezed orange juice, so this may be better to avoid.

Smoothie suggestions

If you are going to mix fruits, try to use the suggestions below or similar fruits because this helps you to reduce the sugar rush. The problem with a natural sugar rush is that you also get a low later on which means that you will be craving sweet foods.

- Half a cup of Strawberries

- Three quarters of a cup of blueberries

- A handful of raspberries

- 1 and a half cups of spinach

This smoothie can be used in the place of a dessert. Remember when you use smoothies that there is a certain amount of calories but they can really help you because the use of fresh fruits will give you added vitamin and minerals.

- Half a cup of Strawberries

- Half a cup of pineapples

- A cup of unsweetened almond milk

Experiment with your smoothies, but mix the types of fruit that you use to get a good balance.

Main Meals

If you are accustomed to eating large meals, you need to get into a new habit. You can eat quite a lot and still lose weight, but it is better if you don't overload your system with too much food at one sitting. Therefore, if you cut back the amount you eat at lunch, you can snack at 3 and then eat again in the evening. If you find that you eat a heavy meal in the evening, try a lighter meal and then a snack a little later on, as long as it is not too close to bedtime.

Your main meals should include a variety of fresh vegetables and also make sure that you look at the list of foods, which are fiber based so that you have a good balance of fiber in your diet. Your main meal can consist of different courses, and there's nothing wrong with having a prawn salad as a starter, followed by a white meat and vegetables, followed by your dessert and the cheese board. The only thing to remember is that smaller portions more frequently are better than loading your system down with too much food at a time.

Desserts

You can have dessert, but you need to be aware of your calorie intake. If, for example, you know that you have eaten heavily for the main meal, use lightweight desserts rather than piling on even more calories and the potential of suffering indigestion. Chew your food well. Take your time and enjoy your meals.

Drink your tea in between meals or after them and space out your tea drinking during the day so that you have finished the bottle of tea by the evening. Alternate tea drinking with water drinking.

Chapter 9: Why Seven Days?

You want to achieve weight loss and you want to see results. The reason that we have suggested a detox of seven days is because this is short enough not to be too much of a task, but it's long enough to help you to change some of your lifestyle habits on a permanent basis. The reason I say this is because on normal diets, as soon as the desired weight loss has happened, people tend to go back to eating their normal diet. The idea of this diet is to educate you about how good you can feel when you use restraint, as well as the obvious benefit of weight loss.

As you get accustomed to wise choices, you will find that you tend to put aside unhealthy foods because you know that your body is thanking you for the detox. You will feel less tired. You won't be constipated and your immune system will be sharper. A lot of the benefits take a couple of days to start being felt so if you only dieted for three days – for example – you may not have really received all the benefits that nettle tea can give you. Thus, we chose seven days because it takes you through all of your lifestyle changes, such as workdays and weekends and if you can eat wisely on these days, then you will find that you can hop onto the detox diet when you feel that your body tells you it needs it.

If you are serious about detoxing your body, you need to give it a week and you should always weigh yourself at the same time every day. Give yourself a start weight so that you have something to aim at and even if some days the weight increases, you may find that the variance in your diet is causing this to happen. Don't be too concerned about it. I would suggest that the best time to weigh yourself is before your evening meal. That way, you have had a little time to burn off your lunch and your afternoon snack.

Avoid packet treats and soda

If you are going to have an afternoon or evening snack, make it nutritious. It is better to eat nuts and fruit than it is to eat a packet of chips. Avoid soda. You should have sufficient drink with your tea and water without introducing more drinks.

Toilet Habits

You may think that you will be going to the toilet more often because of the amount that you are drinking. However, it may surprise you that you don't actually do that apart from being regular at passing stools. This is because the detox is working. It should not cause discomfort and you should try to get into a routine so that you go regularly each day.

Seven days of fitness

Many people are overweight these days and much of this is due to the sedentary lifestyles that people have adopted. It is a good idea to try to get plenty of bodily movement while you are on the detox. This helps the nettle tea to get to where it can do its work quickly and efficiently. If you are accustomed to sitting down after eating, try going for a short walk. If you have a pet, you can use this as an excuse to walk. If you are used to driving to work, park a little further away and try to use the stairs instead of the escalator. Detoxing actually means taking responsibility for the cleansing of your body from the inside, but it doesn't stop there. You need to take responsibility for your fitness and this will also help you to lose even more weight as well as feeling healthier.

At the end of seven days, you will be able to measure the results and should find that these improve the way that you feel. If you want to continue after the seven days, an occasional cup of nettle tea will do you no harm at all. Personally, I have a very strict regime of using nettle tea for one week a month every month. That way, I don't have to worry too much about my body because I know that it hasn't built up enough toxins to worry about it having an effect on my health. The information contained in this book has been backed up by specialists in plant medicine – which has been in use since the Roman times. We now know that the benefits are staggering and as a direct result of your body's metabolism increasing, your body will work better for longer and will digest the food that you eat without the creation of pockets of fat that will eventually add to your waistline size. That's got to be worthwhile.

Chapter 10: A Brief History of Tea

Herbal medicine is certainly nothing new. It is the use of a plant's seed, berries, roots, leaves, bark or flowers for medicinal purpose and it's been used for centuries before the advent of what we all now refer to as modern or conventional medicine—the use of chemically-synthesized ingredients.

In ancient China, green tea was heavily used in to treat feelings of depression and headaches and today, it is popular due to its healing and refreshing properties.

The usage of a tea cleanse diet to detoxify the body is a practice that dates back to an old Indian ritual of physical and spiritual preparation popularly referred to as **Pancha Karma**. Pancha Karma is a branch of Ayurvedic medicine that requires people to undergo spiritual renewal and the severing of negative emotional patterns to prevent diseases.

It involves three stages. The first stage is the preparation phase in which you prepare your body by abstaining from sweet, processed foods and drinks containing caffeine and instead meditate and walk in natural environment taking in the fresh breath of the environment and letting it give you inner calm.

The second stage is referred to as the cleaning stage which the use of laxative to flush away toxins already present in the body.

In the third stage, which is the rejuvenation stage, solid foods are gradually re-introduced into the body. Tea cleanse diet doesn't only have roots in India and China, evidences obtained by researchers have shown this practice to historically practiced by the Egyptians and the Greeks.

Chapter 11: Why Drink Tea?

First and foremost, you must understand that there are different kinds of teas and they vary by origin, color, odor, and their effects on the body. Drinking tea helps in the reduction of cholesterol level and the prevention of diseases like heart diseases, dementia, and cancer.

Very popular types of tea include green tea, black tea, Oolong tea, matcha tea, herbal tea, etc. All Green tea, Black tea, and Oolong are sourced from the same plant, the Camellia Sinensis. Green tea is very useful in burning fat because it contains anti-oxidant features that help increase rate of body metabolism. Green tea also helps the body fight against influenza and common cold.

Here are other benefits you stand to get through a tea cleanse diet:

1. Detoxification

A very good advantage of tea cleansing is that it helps the body in getting rid of excessive waste and toxins that are have accumulated in the body over time. Herbal and green teas naturally assists the body in flushing out many of these toxins. It also helps the body create a healthy blood circulatory system as well as improve metabolism. A lot of detox diets contains herbs, celery, green tea and other low-calorie veggies.

2. Fortified Immune system

Teas contain some active ingredients that keep your lymphatic system healthy and firing on all cylinders. By reducing your sugar, caffeine, and trans-fat consumption and taking a lot of tea, you'll be giving your body a jump in natural energy. Research has also shown that tea drinking can help you reduce significantly your risk of stroke and heart disease, reduce your blood pressure, improve mental performance and give you a boost in energy while still keeping your weight down. For example, the consumption of green tea helps the blood to improve its antioxidant power which protects the Low Density Lipoprotein (LDL) cholesterol particles from oxidation; a pathway to the development of a heart disease. Even though many factors may influence brain health, polyphenols in green tea may help maintain the section of the brain that is responsible for regulating learning and memory.

3. Weight loss

Take a little test and look at the ingredients of most weight-loss supplements that you can find around you. You will discover that majority of those supplements have green tea listed amongst the active ingredients. The reason is not far-fetched. It is simply because green tea increases metabolic rate.

4. Endurance Boost

Teas are great for improving cardiovascular endurance because of its antioxidant constituents (catechins), which increases the body's ability to burn fat and converting it into fuel that can improve the muscle's endurance.

5. Radiation shield

Tea drinking can help protect the body against radiation such as UV-rays. A study found that tea can help shield your skin from cellular degeneration upon exposure to radiation while there's another study that showed that tea drinking can help the skin recover from over sun exposure.

6. Encourages healthy habits

Habits are difficult to change, especially if they are life-long. If you have a knack for sugar, caffeine, fried or crunchy foods, then a tea cleanse diet is what you need to quench those desires. Ordinarily, you can stop consuming unhealthy foods on your own, but you may have limited success doing that and will probably return to your old ways. But by engaging in herbal tea drinking, you will cleanse your body and that will help your body restrain itself and readjust to make healthier food choices.

7. Fights against free radicals

Tea is high in Oxygen Radical Absorbance Capacity (ORAC). This is a technical way of saying that tea drinking helps to remove free radicals, which can cause damage to the DNA since the body on its own cannot totally fight these free radicals. These radicals have been known to cause cancer, heart disease and neurological degeneration.

Chapter 12: Types of Teas and Their Benefits

If you check the shelves of your local store, you will most definitely find different types and brands of teas. But from the perspective of tea purists, the tea you see all around you are not really the 'real' tea. They are just different brews of different herbs I. The real tea are just of four types: Black tea, green tea, White tea and Oolong and they all come from the plant, the Camellia sinensis. Yes, the same plant which originates from China and some parts of India. The resulting differences in their characteristic appearance, flavor and health benefits is due to the cultivation and processing of the plants' leaves. Let's dive down a bit into these types of teas so you can understand them better.

1. Green tea:

This is arguably the most famous tea in the world. It is processed by steaming the leaves of the Camellia sinensis and has a very high level of epigallocatechin-3-gallate (EGCG); an antioxidant that prevents the growth of cancers, clogging of the blood vessels, and reduces the risk of stroke and brain disorders like Parkinson's and Alzheimer diseases.

2. Black tea:

This is processed by fermenting the leaves of the Camellia Sinensis and has a very high concentration of caffeine. It has been reported that regular ingestion of black tea helps reduce the risk of lung damage that may arise from being exposed to smoke from cigarettes.

3. White tea:

This doesn't undergo any processing. Hence, it is regarded as the purest of teas. It is very rich in antioxidants and the results of a study has shown that it is the most effective of all teas when it comes to its anti-cancer properties.

4. Oolong tea:

Oolong teas undergo partial fermentation and makes use of an additional shaking process that releases additional flavors. Oolong can vary in color from dark green to black. This combination of partial fermentation and bruising is responsible for its flowery and earthy flavor. It has less oxidants and higher caffeine content than green tea.

Finally, because of its popular usage and advantage, it is important that we discuss herbal teas

5. Herbal tea:

Herbal teas aka tisanes can be said to be any beverage made from the infusion or decoction of herbs, spices, or other medicinal parts of a plant in hot water and usually doesn't contain caffeine. They are different from white, green, black, and oolong because they are not made from the plant **Camellia sinensis** and which contains caffeine. Herbal teas can be made hot or cold.

Chapter 13: Brewing Your Tea

Now that we've discussed the health benefits of teas and the different types that are available to you, let's delve into how you can brew your own tea. Before we go further, it is important to have it in mind that there are different ways to brew your tea and each brewing method has an effect on the functionality or health benefits of each tea.

You'd probably heard of infusions, decoctions, and tinctures and don't know what they really mean or how they are prepared. You are in luck as this will be broken down for you. Infusions, decoctions, and tinctures are all different ways of extracting the chemical constituents of teas from the plant material through the use of a solvent such as water or alcohol. When you engage in tea preparation, infusions, and decoctions, you are using water; a universal solvent to extract all of the plant's constituents like alkaloids, glycosides, saponins, flavonoids, tannins, mucilage, polysaccharides, vitamins, minerals, small amounts of volatile oils except resins. This solvent base is then consumed making it easy for the body to absorb those constituents. This knowledge will guide you in getting a particular action from a certain herb because of its constituents.

Infusion

You can brew a tea or make an infusion by pouring water over a soft herb such as the flowers, stem or leaves of the plant you intend to use and allowing it to steep for a certain period of time. To make an infusion, you will need

- Clean, cold water

- Approx. 1-2 teaspoon of the dried tea to make a serving

- Boil your water and pour over your herbs.

- Allow the mixture to steep for about 10-20 minutes while covered.

- Strain the water off the herbs and serve.

If your plan is to make a medicinal infusion, your best bet is to use more herbs per cup of water and increase the steeping time to about an hour. Also, note that infusions relatively do not last long so ensure to consume within a day of preparation. You should note that different teas require different brewing time. That is to say, delicate teas like green tea require shorter brewing time compared to black teas and fermented pu-erh teas which thrive on lengthier infusion period.

Decoctions

Decoctions are generally prepared by simmering harder herbs (roots, nuts, seeds, barks) over low heat for a specified period of time. To get more usefulness out of the herbs, it is advised that you crush the herbs to reduce the surface area which will make the extraction easier. Ground herbs is also available, but they have a lower shelf-life than whole herbs. Generally decoctions are stronger than infusions. To make a decoction, you can follow this step.

- Get clean, cold water

- Use approximately 1/3 ounce of the crush dried herb per cup of water. You can use fresh herbs too but note that if you are using fresh herbs, you will have to double the measurement.

- Boil your water and add the herbs you intend to use

- Turn down the heat and keep it covered. The reason you should cover it up is that an important constituent such as essential oils can be lost through evaporation.

- Simmer the mixture for about 30 minutes if the size of the herbs you are using is small. But if you are processing bigger herb sizes such as barks or root, you should employ a longer simmering time.

- When you are done, remove from heat, strain and serve. You don't necessarily need to serve immediately. You can steep for a longer period of time if you want.

Tinctures

Tinctures are also good herbal extracts that employs the use of alcohol, glycerin, or vinegar. To make a tincture, follow these steps. It should be noted that tinctures are generally stronger than infusions and decoctions.

- Finely-divide the herbs you want to use (bark, roots, etc)

- Get a clean glass jar

- Keep the herbs in the glass jar and pour alcohol in it until the herbs are completely submerged in it.

- Cover up the mixture and note the date it was prepared

- Every day, shake the mixture for the first week and allow it brew for about 4 weeks

- At the end of the stipulated period, pour the tincture into a bottle and serve

Chapter 14: General Guidelines

Brewing a delicious cup of tea which is rich and healthy requires the right combinations of tea leaves, the quantity of water used, temperature of water, duration of infusion, and even the brewing container.

Temperature

Boiled water is commonly used but some constituents may better be extracted using cold water, that's why it's best to know which plant you are using and what you want to extract before you decide on the temperature of water to use.

Quantity of herbs

The quantity of herbs in a preparation sure makes a lot of difference as you may have noticed. Normally, to make a serving of tea, you might need 1-3 tsp. off herb per 8oz. cup. To make an infusion or decoction, you might need 1 oz. of dried herb per 4 cups of water and 1/3 cup of dried herbs to 4 cups of water. However, this is not a universal standard as you are free to make your own choice depending on the value you want to get out of it. As you will observe, teas use less herbs and therefore have a light taste in flavor whereas infusions and decoctions use more water and have stronger flavor.

Steep time

Real tea (teas that contain actual tea leaves) generally have a steeping time in the range of 3-5 minutes while some herbal teas are steeped around 10-15 minutes. Depending on how strong you want your infusions to be, steeping time actually be varied. Common steeping time can range from 30 minutes to 12 hours.

Brewing material

While it may seem like an unimportant factor at first in the grand scheme of things, the brewing material plays a role in the quality of the tea infusion. It is important that you carefully consider the type of tea and the temperature at which it is to be brewed. Materials made from Iron or Chinese yixing are excellent when it comes to retaining heat over a relatively long period of time while materials like glass or porcelain aren't that effective because they tend to lose heat faster than metals. Therefore, iron and similar metals are good materials for brewing teas that require relatively high temperatures like black tea or yixing. While a material like porcelain will be just good enough to brew teas like Green and White teas.

General brewing information for some selected teas

Type of Tea: **White**

Amount: 2-3 teaspoon

Time of Infusion: **3 minutes**

Temperature: 176° - 185° F

Type of Tea: **Green**

Amount: 1-2 teaspoon

Time of Infusion: **1-2 minutes**

Temperature: 158° - 176° F

Type of Tea: **Oolong**

Amount: 2-3 teaspoon

Time of Infusion: **2-3 minutes**

Temperature: 185° - 203° F

Type of Tea: **Black**

Amount: 1-2 teaspoon

Time of Infusion: **2-3 minutes**

Temperature: **203° F**

Type of Tea: **Pu-erh**

Amount: 1-2 teaspoon

Time of Infusion: **3 minutes**

Temperature: **212° F**

Type of Tea: **Herbal**

Amount: 1-2 teaspoon

Time of Infusion: **3 minutes**

Temperature: **212° F**

Chapter 15: Selecting a Sweetener

Understanding the fact that some teas have a very bitter taste, for example black tea, makes the choice of using a sweetener necessary. Normally, it is advised that you drink your tea without any additive or sweetener, that way you get the most benefits out of your tea in terms of the health implications on your body. However, if you cannot stomach the bitterness and instead will like to alter the taste of your tea, you will be left with two options of sweeteners which are:

1. White Sugar

2. Honey

Essentially, both are sugars when you consider their chemistry.

White sugar comprises of about 50% fructose and 50% glucose. Both sugars are chemically bounded to form sucrose aka white sugar. Ingesting white sugar means your body will have to do a job of breaking down the sucrose to get the glucose it needs since the body burns glucose to fuel its operations. The breakdown of this white sugar then leads to an increase in blood glucose level. A tablespoon of sugar gives about 49 calories and 15 grams of carbohydrate per tablespoon.

Honey too contains sugar, but in a lesser amount compared to white sugar since it contains about 30%

glucose and less than 40% fructose, trace amounts of vitamins and minerals and other useful anti-oxidants. Unlike white sugar where the constituent molecules are chemically bonded together and your body has to do the extra job of separating the glucose it needs, the sugars in honey are available in free form for your body to use immediately. This means the body doesn't have to work itself to get the fuel it needs from honey. This is also why honey tastes sweeter than sugar since fructose (which is sweeter than glucose) is freely available. Honey has a bit higher density than sugar contains, about 68 calories and 17.2 grams of carbohydrate per tablespoon.

By now, it should be clear that honey has more health benefits than white sugar. But for the sake of clarity, the benefits will be highlighted below.

1. Honey has other constituents like vitamins, anti-oxidants, and starch that provides the body with additional benefits while white sugar is essential glucose and fructose.

2. The body absorbs honey better than it does sugar.

3. Honey has a lower glycemic index (GI) compared to white sugar and thus poses a lesser risk of causing diabetes.

4. Honey contains more calories per tablespoon than sugar. Hence, it is more energy-giving than sugar.

5. If you are watching your weight, honey is a smarter choice for you

6. Honey tastes far better than sugar even though both are sweet hence its use in the food industry as flavor.

Chapter 16: Using Tea Cleanse For Weight Loss

According to the results of a study published by the Institute of Physiology at the University of Fribourg in Switzerland, EGCG, a component found in green tea plus caffeine improves thermogenesis (the generation of body heat due to normal digestion process, absorption, and food metabolism) by about 84%. The result also goes on to state that green tea increases norepinephrine, the chemical which burns fat to provide your give your body the "fight or flight" response that is typical of adrenaline.

Even though some researchers don't totally agree that tea is the "holy grail" of weight loss, what every weight loss expert will agree on is the fact that tea or water drinking works more effectively than chewing candy bars or sipping sodas frequently. Since tea and water consumption aids the process of digestion, it will help with a reduction in the waistline. Whether or not tea drinking is charming, it is a good idea when trying to reduce your weight.

The first step to using tea to lose weight is to choose a tea based on its effectiveness. Green, white, and oolong are considered very effective, black tea is considered moderately effective, and decaffeinated or herbal teas are considered good enough.

Secondly, you must make tea drinking a daily ritual. You can't be doing it intermittently, you must be consistent. Create a tea-time in your schedule and make sure you stick to it. Take a cup of strong tea in the morning and another in the afternoon, then drink another less effective tea like herbal tea during bed time since they are decaffeinated and won't cause you to lose sleep. Ensure that you brew your tea in advance so you will always have a continuous supply.

Thirdly, even though we discussed sweeteners earlier, ensure that you do not add anything to your tea. Milk and sugar will affect any benefit the tea will offer you. Whenever you feel the urge to eat, try to quench that feeling by taking a cup of tea to regulate your metabolism. Whenever you feel need to eat something sugary, make a nice brew of tea to take away the hunger.

To continue to sustain the momentum and keep yourself going, it's highly important that you settle on a drink that you really like and enjoy. Some teas could be very bitter and unpleasant to taste. Others may possess pungent and repulsive smell and there are many others that are really good for beginners.

You will hear a lot about diet teas. Many taste very similar to herbal teas but may contain ingredients that have a laxative effect on the body. That means there is a caveat here. Don't excessively consume these teas in moderation. Yes, you want to reduce your weight but you also want to do it the healthy way and not become hospitalized in the process. Watch out for ingredient like senna, agarwood, rhubarb root or castor oil. One cup of diet tea is enough per day unless you want to deal with vomiting, nausea, diarrhea, abdominal cramps, etc. Therefore before you buy your tea, look at the ingredient label very carefully, if sugar or a sweetener has been added, don't buy it. However, you find that some green teas are flavored, but as long as you can, stay off teas which don't have natural ingredients.

Make your tea easy to brew and constantly available

A major reason a lot of people find it hard to follow a particular weight loss program even a program as easy as a tea cleanse diet is that the tools to really accomplishing them are not easily within reach. So to make brewing your tea very easy, buy your electric teakettle and put it in a very easy to reach place. Brewing tea is very simple. Fill the electric kettle with water and boil the water to the desired temperature. When this is achieved, pour the water into a cup and brew the tea by adding several tea bags to the hot water while giving it 2 to 3 minutes for all the useful constituents to be fully extracted. To make tea brewing easier throughout the day since the goal is to lose weight, ensure that you have a continuous supply of water all through the day, for this, you can get a thermos flask.

Start your day with a cup of tea in the morning instead of whatever it is you are used to. Take it without any "additive" like cream or sugar since the addition of cream reduces the efficacy of flavonoids; the constituent of tea responsible for fat removal.

Stay away from soda during lunch or dinner since it is a culprit when it comes to weight gain. You can opt for sugar-free iced tea instead. Iced tea is very good if your choice is a blend of tea with a touch of caffeine. Much of the trick behind a tea cleanse diet is that you won't be taking anything else instead. Tea has low calories and will prevent you from consuming other things that will ramp up your calories.

If you spend over 6 hours at the office, then it make sense that you have your tea stash somewhere in your drawer along with a fancy mug and a thermos flask that holds previously boiled water. You can even make it social by making an extra cup of tea for a friend or coworker on a frequent basis. If you have friends that are also trying to reduce their waist lines through a tea cleanse diet, then that's great. The more the merrier.

By dinner time, drink a cool glass of tea. Doing this will mean that you will be less hungry for food. That doesn't mean a healthy dinner doesn't make sense or that you should starve yourself. But since the plan is to reduce weight and cold tea gets heated up by the body which makes it burn extra calories resulting in weight loss, which would you prefer?

Just before going to bed, regardless of whether you have plans for your weight, drink up a cup of herbal tea. This will help you relax your brain and body.

Eat a healthy diet for your weight loss program

You should keep in mind that the best weight loss diet still requires that you eat healthy food. Tea drinking for weight loss is good but combining it with a healthy diet is better. Drink your tea with whole grains, fruits, and low-fat dairy products. And since you'll be brewing your tea yourself, why not cook your own food? This way you decide exactly what you are eating in terms of nutrients, taste, and form. Therefore, it's best to avoid eat-outs while reducing the consumption of processed and canned foods.

Create a variety of tea drinks

It certainly won't help drinking the same type of tea for an extended period of time, the same way you won't want to eat the same meal for the rest of the year. In the end, you will get tired of it. Therefore, change your routine, mix your tea and try different teas, flavors, and enhancements. You can stock your cupboard with different varieties of teas, add honey to your brewed tea occasionally, or even try a splash of lemon to help your tea cleanse weight loss program going. Here are some very interesting tea varieties to check out and they are all good for weight loss:

Star anise tea: improves digestion and can help relax stomach upset

Peppermint tea: Improves appetite and aids digestion

Rose tea: helps keep constipation away and is rich in vitamins

Chapter 17: The 30-Day Weight Loss Challenge

To help you get on top of your game with a tea cleanse diet that's effective, it's important that you create a structured program that is going to allow you keep all the tea cleanse diet principles in mind. The result you will get if you keep to this program will be tremendous. Here are some great tips to help you get started right away.

Get a scale

The first step is determining if you are under, over, or of regular weight. If you find out that you are overweight then proceed to the next step.

Quit the blame game

Cast aside whatever negative feeling you have about your weight. It hasn't helped anybody and it won't help you. Going forward, don't put unnecessary pressure on yourself but instead have a positive outlook about yourself and believe that your plan will yield fruits.

Start cutting away sugar

There is sugar everywhere and you should stop consuming them.

Set goals that are SMART

At the end of 30 days, you should have a particular weight you want to cut off. Your goal should be **Specific** not wild. It should be **Measurable**; you should see how many pounds you are losing per week. It should also be **Achievable**; don't think you can lose 100 pounds in a week by tea drinking only. It must be **Realistic and Time-bound.**

Get your tea brewing tools

Purchase an electric kettle, a set of mugs, tea spoon and a vacuum flask so you can have a continuous supply of tea all day.

Select your tea

A lot has been said about this earlier. You have the choice of green, white, black, oolong, and herbal teas. Their effectiveness varies as much as their taste. Green and white teas are the most effective while herbal teas or tisanes are the least effective of the teas.

Brew your first tea

For a start, you can brew white or green teas first as they are relatively faster to prepare compared to herbal teas. They also have great tastes too. Drink your tea very early in the morning, afternoon, and evening.

Try a different type of tea

You are trying a different type of tea because you want to vary the taste of your tea and you are trying to find out which is best for you not just for the fun of changing teas.

Settle for the type of tea you want and continue drinking

By day 9, you should have settled for the type of tea that fits your weight loss plan and that's equally sustainable in terms of taste, affordability, and ease of acquisition.

Intensify your efforts and stay away from fattening foods

Now that you've found a tea you are willing to take on a regular basis, the next step is to start taking it on a regular basis! Don't miss a schedule. For best results, you are expected to drink at least 2-3 cups of tea every day.

Check your metrics

Has there been a change in your weight for the past 11 days? If there is, note and record it in a journal. Your achievement should be measured and celebrated. Continue doing this for the next 9 days and note any change in your waistline

Overall assessment

To be candid, you may not get the kind of result you want immediately. This may be due to the nature of your body, the choice of tea, the frequency of consumption amongst other factors. Most experts will also agree that losing weight is harder than gaining weight, so if you haven't seen any significant change after a few days of engaging in tea cleanse diet, don't be alarmed. Just continue to follow this guide and intensify your efforts.

FAQ: Frequently Asked Questions about tea cleanse diet

Q: Does drinking tea has side effects?

A: A lot of herbal drinks are safe for consumption, however, there are herbs that have toxic or allergenic effects. For example, Comfrey, which contains alkaloids and can cause permanent liver damage with chronic use.

Q: How long will the tea cleanse diet take before I start seeing the results?

A: The duration varies from person to person and is dependent on the choice of tea and consistency of use. However, if you use a strong tea and drink a cup of tea about three times daily, you should start seeing the results between 1-3 months.

Part 2

Introduction

There are so many kinds of diet regimens sprouting up every now and then. Some involve vegetables, others fruits, and of course, there are a whole lot of those green juice diets, too.

But did you know that you could actually go on a Tea Cleanse diet?

Yes! In fact, various kinds of teas have different kinds of uses—and with the help of this book, you'll learn how following a tea cleanse diet can help you lose weight and rinse away toxins, what the best kinds of tea to drink are, and more!

Read this book now and lose weight in just 3 weeks—all thanks to tea.

Thanks again for downloading this book, I really hope you enjoy it!

Chapter 1: How Tea Helps You Lose Weight

So, you're probably wondering how exactly does tea help you lose weight, and how it detoxifies the body, right ?

EGCG Metabolizes Fat

Well, the thing with tea is that it naturally metabolizes fat, because Epigalocatechin Gallate, also known as EGCG, or fat burning hormones, are activated when tea is broken down in the digestive system, and when it makes its way to the bloodstream.

EGCG is a polyphenol that works the same way as most dietary supplements—and yes, you have it in your body, and you only need tea to activate it! Studies show that not only does EGCG helps you lose weight, it also aids in the prevention of cancer, HIV, and other diseases, as well.

Another amazing thing about EGCG is the fact that it breaks down Noripinepherine.

What Is Noripinepherine?

Don't mind the complicated name; Noripinepherine are neurotransmitters that are important in the aspect of cognitive alertness. This means that it could push fat cells to break fat down, and release it to the bloodstream as energy, instead of just keeping it in the stomach, and allow it to put more weight on you.

It Has Caffeine, Too!

Caffeine is not all that bad. In fact, caffeine found in tea is definitely a whole lot less than what's found in coffee. Tea only has around 400 milligrams of caffeine. As it is a stimulant, caffeine helps one lose weight by:

1. Suppressing the appetite. It helps you feel satiated for a long time so you wouldn't think about eating over and over again. When the appetite is suppressed, the body only gets to take in a few amount of calories, and;

2. **It burns calories.** This happens by means of thermogenesis. Basically, thermogenesis is how energy is generated through body heat, activated by tea, and other food sources.

You see, these elements found in tea make it the fat-burning drink that it is. Not only that, studies also show that tea aids in exercise regimens—making them more effective and easy to do, as well!

Rest, Reduce, Rebuild

The main principle of the tea cleanse diet is Rest, Reduce, and Rebuild. With the help of tea, you'll easily be able to chew your food (more on this later), which means that metabolism would not suffer.

According to Roni DeLuz, a naturopathic doctor, a tea cleanse session should last for 3 weeks, or 21 days. There should be a week-long cleanse for the first 3 weeks, and weekend detox on the next couple of weeks, just so you could maintain your figure and so your health would not suffer.

It doesn't mean that you cannot eat anything else, though. Around 32 to 40 ounces of tea per day is good, combined with 40 to 48 ounces of water, 32 ounces of berry or vegetable juices, and 16 ounces of vegetable-based soup.

You can also add the following to your diet:

Purple cabbage, tomatoes, green vegetables, summer squash, sweet potatoes, radish, onions, beet, kale, eggplant, collard greens, celery, cucumbers, carrot, pureed, powdered, or juiced garlic, lean beef, fish, lean chicken, lean turkey, yogurt, tofu, lima means, non-dairy milk

And, make sure to avoid the following:

Processed food, high-fat meat and eggs, coffee, salt & alcohol

Determine Real from Emotional Hunger

The best part about the tea cleanse diet is that it actually helps you determine real from emotional hunger.

Emotional hunger happens when you feel a sudden surge of hunger (even though you have just eaten moments ago), when you have certain food cravings, when you keep eating even when you're already full, and when you feel unsatisfied, no matter how much you have eaten.

But, with the help of the tea cleanse diet, this will be prevented from happening because you'd always be satiated and so, you'd be able to experience real hunger as you should.

Real hunger happens when hunger starts to arise gradually, when you do not feel the need to easily be full, when you're open to a lot of food options, and when you get to that state where you feel like you're full and you feel good at it, instead of feeling guilty or ashamed.

And that's so much better, right?

Chapter 2: Detoxifying With Tea

While you may lose weight with the help of tea, it also detoxifies the body, which makes the regimen all the more effective.

There are two major ways in which tea detoxifies the body, and these are:

Refreshing the Body

The first part of the Tea Cleanse Diet is called Refresh. This should be done in the morning (you'll learn more about the schedule in the next chapter), but mainly, Refresh should be done in the morning.

With this part of the detox program, vitamins and electrolytes that have been lost in the body are replaced. Take note that it is important to go on this process first, or else no detoxification would happen!

For this, you can try:

1. **Matcha.** Matcha is one of the most popular teas out there and is definitely one of the most nutritious. It burns calories, boosts metabolism, filled with fiber that drives toxins away, and is also packed with antioxidants that keep the skin radiant and young-looking. Not only that, it also contains essential

vitamins such as magnesium, zinc, selenium, and Vitamin C that could replace the ones you have lost. Matcha also enhances the mood, so drinking it in the morning could really help you feel better and more energetic throughout the day!

2. **Barley Grass.** Barley Grass kills free radicals that could destroy the body, and is also instrumental in the prevention of gout and rheumatoid arthritis. Barley also increases the production of fat-burning enzymes that could of course help you lose fat. Barley Grass also contains a lot of essential vitamins such as folic and pantothenic acid, B Vitamins, calcium, and beta-carotene, and is an amazing source of fiber!

3. **Acai Berry.** Acai Berry is considered a superfood because of its high antioxidant content that helps refresh the body in a holistic manner. Acai also has a lot of heart-healthy fats, too!

4. **Ginseng.** Ginseng is an amazing immune system booster. It lowers blood and cholesterol levels, treats sexual dysfunction and diabetes, and eases stress. You can use both Asian and American Ginseng.

5. **Spirulina.** Sure, you may feel like Spirulina is way out of your league as it is freshwater algae, but you'll surely love the benefits!

Colon Cleanse

The next part of the diet is the Colon Cleanse, which means that you have to work on strengthening the body. This is important because unhealthy colon could be susceptible to diseases.

For this, you have to use Senna Leaf as base.

What Is Senna Leaf?

Senna Leaf is a natural laxative that prevents and treats constipation and irritable bowel syndrome. This means that detoxification would come easy, and so does weight loss.

Since Senna Leaf has quite a strong taste, it is important that you blend it with other types of tea so you'd easily be able to drink it, and so cleansing the colon would become easier. You can blend Senna Leaf with the following:

1. **Dried Orange Peel.** One of the most soothing natural products that you can use is Dried Orange Peel, which not only smells good, it also clears respiratory tracts, and keeps you safe from diseases! Surely, it'll mask the taste of Senna Leaf without juicing it out of nutrients—and that's why it's good for you!

2. Dandelion. Dandelion is one of the most powerful tonics as it improves liver function. Not only that, it also prevents and treats kidney stones, gall stones, and has a lot of anti-bacterial properties, and is also a natural laxative that balances the microbiome, stimulates appetite, and promotes digestion. It is

also said that Dandelion could help prevent diabetes and cancer, and also has a lot of antioxidants that slow down the aging process.

3. **Nettle Leaf.** Nettle Leaf is a natural diuretic and astringent, and one that could reverse the effects of Urinary Tract problems. Studies show that Nettle Leaf could also prevent and treat alopecia (hair loss), and well as joint ailments!

4. Lemon Grass. Yes, lemon grass is not just something that could add more aroma to your dishes, it's also quite beneficial because it can be used in aromatherapy. It prevents high blood pressure, convulsions, pain, count, and joint ailments, as well as muscle pain!

5. **Licorice Root.** You also need some Licorice Root in your diet because it rids the colon of toxins, and could also prevent inflammation of the stomach. Licorice Root could also prevent and treat food poisoning, It also treats bronchitis, cough, colic, stomach ulcers, and heartburn—so you always have to keep it in handy!

Chapter 3: The Schedule

As you may have read earlier, there is a certain schedule that you have to adhere to, so that the diet would really work. You do not have to worry because the schedule is quite simple and you'd easily be able to get through it!

In the Morning

Again, Refresh should be done in the morning. To aid you with this, it would be good if you could boil some water and wake yourself up first by mixing tea with lemon slices, lemon juice, or ginger. This'll wake you up, and start the process of enhancing metabolism right away!

Time for Refresh

Now is the real time for Refresh. Take note that this should be done after drinking your warm-up drink (the one you made earlier). Choose either Matcha, Acai, Ginseng, Barley, or Spirulina. You could add these with other ingredients, but make sure they would be the base. This'll give you a boost of energy that you'll need throughout the day!

Drink Other Kinds of Tea

In the next few chapters, you'll find out which teas you can drink throughout the day!

Colon Cleanse

And finally, shortly before going to bed, make tea that's based on the colon cleanse ingredients you learned about in an earlier chapter!

Follow this schedule for at least 1 to 3 weeks before taking some rest! Anyway, that is the goal of this book to make you lose 15 lbs in just 3 weeks and that's what you'll be able to do!

Chapter 4: 1st Week- Teas That Boost Metabolism

Not all teas are created the same. In this chapter, you'll learn all about teas that easily boost Metabolism more than others! Surely, these will help you lose weight fast!

Try these on the first week of the diet!

Star Anise Tea

Native to China, Star Anise treats stomach upset and diarrhea—and also helps suppress the appetite!

To get maximum effects, steep a Star Anise pod for at least 10 minutes. Feel free to blend it with other ingredients or teas because drinking it alone might be a little too bitter for your taste.

Peppermint Tea

You know what's great about Peppermint Tea? Well, it actually helps your body gain more control when it comes to the things you eat. It helps you keep satiated, and taps EGCG to do its job, therefore enhancing metabolism!

You can make peppermint tea by using the leaves of the peppermint plant. Use either fresh or dried leaves and steep for at least 4 to 5 minutes.

Yerba Mate

Good Cholesterol Levels are stimulated with the help of Yerba Mate. Enzymes that break down bad cholesterol are tapped with the help of polyphenols and antioxidants that are found in Yerba Mate.

Make some by using a coffee grinder or by steeping the tea in squash gourd!

Porangaba Tea

Mostly found in South America, Porangaba is known as Brazil's special weight loss potion. It has just the right amount of caffeine that could hasten metabolic rate and prevent fat from ruining the body.

More so, Porangaba suppresses the appetite, but does not destroy the organs as it is a natural diuretic. Drink some 30 minutes before each meal and you're all set!

Rose Tea

Rose Tea boosts metabolism as it contains a combination of Vitamins A, B3, C, D, and E. Not only that, it also keeps the body safe from infections, prevents constipation, and is highly therapeutic.

Use petals and buds to make tea, but make sure to clean the petals first with the help of boiling water. Steep for 2 to 3 minutes.

Not only does it smell good, it actually tastes great, too!

Feiyan Tea

Fat that is accumulated by the body could be reduced with the help of Feiyan Tea.

You see, this tea is made of a combination of plants, such as jasmine, lotus, and vegetable sponge that contain no chemical elements. This means that there would be no side effects, and that you can lose up to 8 lbs in the first week of the diet alone, especially if you drink this on the first night of the diet itself.

Not only does it boost metabolism, it detoxifies the body, too!

Oolong Tea

More than 150% of fat is burned, and metabolism is enhanced substantially with Oolong Tea!

Aside from enhancing metabolism, Oolong Tea also prevents the body from absorbing more fat than it can handle. In just 2 weeks, fat is blocked by up to 50% already, thanks to the natural oxidation process!

Oolong also increases the body's Plasma Adiponectin Levels that are responsible for protecting the body against Obesity.

To make Tea this you simply pre-heat your tea mug or pot by pouring a little amount of hot water into the mug. When the mug is warm simply pour out the boiling water and measure approximately 1-2 tablespoons of Oolong Tea, add that amount to the pre-heated mug along with more boiling water then cover with a small saucer and steep for up to 5 minutes. Make sure to constantly taste it to check if it's up to your standard.

You can either make this in a matter of 5 to 30 minutes; the longer, the more the flavor is maximized!

Chapter 5: 2nd Week: Fat-Blocking Teas

On the 2nd week of the diet, you should drink more of those teas that block fat. Not only that, it's best if you could choose teas that also reverse fat and turn them into energy instead—and you'll find all those teas right here!

White Tea

White Tea is the type of tea that's naturally sun-dried, which makes it full of anti-oxidants. The compounds found in White Tea are then able to block the formation of fat cells, as well as break fat down and turn it into energy instead.

Its antioxidants, meanwhile, are able to trigger fat release from the cells and help the liver turn said fat into energy, which, of course, is good for the body!

Japanese Matcha Tea

You know, learning about tea ceremony isn't just about appreciating art. It's also about knowing that Japanese Tea is actually helpful in the sense that it increases thermogenesis (the use of heat to break fat down, and turn it into energy). From 8 to 10%, thermogenesis reaches a 35 to 48% high! It lowers the amount of bad cholesterol, leaving you healthy and protected from heart diseases, too!

Green Tea

Of course, it all starts with Green Tea!

It's so popular that in fact, it's already known as a post-workout staple. The thing about Green Tea is that it's anti-oxidant features easily break down fat that soon boosts energy and hastens the metabolic rate. This way, even if you're not overly active, you can be sure that fat will still be burned—and that you'd lose weight in no time!

Green Tea also rehydrates the body and generally improves immunity, as well!

Rooibos

The best thing about Rooibos tea is that it inhibits fat cell formation. You see, when there are no fat cells, there's also a very low chance that you'd gain lots of fat, in the first place. By drinking Rooibos tea, you'd get to prevent fat cell formation by up to 22%!

Aside from that, Rooibos also prevents stress, thanks to its unique combination of flavonoids. This way, one's hunger is also suppressed—which leads to fat-burning, as well.

Barberry

Meanwhile, there's also a tea called Barberry—which is amazing because it prevents fat cells from growing larger.

Barberry is a tea made from the Barberry Shrub, which is naturally known to prevent weight gain. This also happens even when one is on a high-fat diet.

More so, Barberry also aids in the development of Insulin Resistance—so it's safe to say that it's good for Diabetics, too. Barberry could also increase your energy levels—and when your energy levels are high, it means that you can do a lot in just a short time. When you're active, you prevent fat from taking over your body—and that's definitely a good thing!

Black Tea

While Barberry prevents fat cells from growing larger, Black Tea is responsible for reducing fat storage hormones in the body by decreasing cortisol levels. Cortisol is responsible for bad cholesterol and fat formation, and when that is shut down, it's easy to say that you'd lose fat in your body, too.

It's best to drink black tea when you are stressed because it's also during that time that adrenaline is able to break fat down, and release fat into your system to turn them into energy.

When Adrenaline and Cortisol work together, the body is able to break more fat down—and in turn, prevent the body from consuming more calories, too!

Pu-erh (Fermented Green Tea)

This tea is the kind that's fermented and then rolled into blocks, which could lower triglyceride compounds. These triglycerides are basically a dangerous kind of fat that's found in one's blood.

Aside from that, Pu-erh also lowers the amount of abdominal fat, even in high-fat diets—which is definitely a good thing!

Chapter 6: 3rd Week: Detoxifying Teas

When you've reached the 3rd week of the diet, it's important to flush toxins away continually, and not only that, you also have to aid it with proper elimination techniques in the following chapter, too!

Here are the teas first.

Cayenne Pepper Tea

Since it is naturally spicy, you can expect cayenne pepper tea to curb your appetite, with the help of capsaicin, and also to flush those toxins while elevating your mood.

Aside from being a good detox aid, it also energizes you a whole lot—making it one of the best teas you can keep!

If you feel like it's a little too hot for you, you could always drink it with lemon slices!

Burdock Root Tea

While not as popular as its contemporaries, Burdock Root can detoxify a lot by being a liver tonic. A highly functioning liver regulates digestive processes, which means that there would be less toxic buildup in your digestive tract. Burdock also purifies the blood and strengthens the immune system—and when holistic healing is promoted, you know you're drinking a good thing!

Cilantro Tea

Cilantro not only spices up your dishes, you could also use it for detoxification purposes!

The thing with cilantro is that it breaks down food so nutrients would easily be released without disrupting your digestive processes. Cilantro is also considered to be highly curative!

Chicory Tea

By drinking chicory tea, it's like you're hitting two birds with one stone because it not only cleanses the body, it also hastens metabolic rate, too.

It's best to drink chicory tea before a meal because it could get digestive juices going, which would then be responsible for the easy breakdown of food. This tea also helps you get all the nutrients you can get from what you have been eating.

Fenugreek Tea

It's best to drink Fenugreek tea when you're feeling a little under the weather and you feel like your digestive system is suffering. It helps keep you from getting bloated, and also helps prevent indigestion from happening.

Inflammation is reduced and high blood pressure is prevented—what more could you ask for?

Ginger Tea

Ginger is considered to be one of the highest cleansing teas out there. Sure, the taste may be a bit sharp, but it's so beneficial, so it really does not matter anymore. Besides, you could always tame it down with the help of lemon slices, you know?

Garlic Tea

Garlic may also prove to be somehow challenging for you to drink, but the thing with it is that it strengthens the body's detoxification process, so even without it, your body would already be able to flush those toxins away!

Garlic also strengthens the immune system and protects you against a lot of diseases, making life even better for you!

Gymnema Sylvestre Tea

This is a Chinese herb that is known for being able to regulate blood glucose levels, and could also reverse the effect of digestive disorders.

More so, it also cleanses the liver and the colon—and makes sure that you are protected against diabetes!

Guduchi Tea

Guduchi has amazing restorative properties that improves organ function and also keeps the skin glowing and healthy at all times!

Milk Thistle Tea

Milk Thistle could help your liver work the best way it could!

You see, detox diets work best when you have something that could really keep the liver safe, and make sure that it does its job of producing the right amount of digestive juices. Milk Thistle regulates digestive processes, too!

Manjistha Tea

Did you know that in order to eliminate toxins, you should also take care of your skin? Well, this is because the skin is the body's largest organ so if you do not take care of it, it wouldn't be able to help the liver in flushing those toxins away.

Manjistha has a lot of medicinal properties, especially for menstruating women. It's best for menstruating women to take this to help keep them calm during that dreaded time of the month, so they could get rid of more toxins and keep their bodies safe!

Red Clover Tea

Red Clover Tea is able to fight free radicals because it contains a lot of antioxidants, and also makes sure that your body would not play host to organisms and parasites that could cause diseases. Always go for organic red clover tea!

Turmeric Tea

Turmeric tea breaks toxins down and flushes them away for good. It also helps the liver produce more bile so that your body would be clean at all times, and so digestive processes would easily be regulated.

Triphala Tea

Triphala treats constipation stimulates bowel movements, which means that your colon would be healthy and clean. It's also important to take care of the colon because if you don't, it could reintroduce those toxins back again—and that's not what you want to happen.

Yellow Dock Tea

Yellow Dock takes care of both the colon and the liver, which means that toxins are easily eliminated, and digestion is improved—definitely making you feel like your best self ever!

Wormwood Tea

And finally, don't forget Wormwood Tea.

This helps the liver produce more bile, and makes sure that digestive processes would not be stagnant. It's also best to drink this daily, even after the 3 weeks of the diet!

Chapter 7: Enhance The Process

As previously mentioned, you'll also learn how to make sure that the 3rd week of the diet works. This could be done by means of enhancing the elimination process. Here's what you have to do:

1. **Drink enough water.** It's not only the liver and kidneys that you should think of; you have to give your kidney the time of day, too! Make sure that while on the tea cleanse diet, you have to go to the bathroom to pee at least once every hour, and that you drink 6 to 8 glasses of water a day. It's always best to stay hydrated!

2. **Boost Circulation**. In order to easily turn fat into energy, you do have to boost circulation. Do so by exercising. You see, you do have to take care of your lymph nodes by making sure lymphatic fluid flows steadily—and deep-breathing exercises as well as jump-roping could help you out with this. It would be nice if you'd find time to laugh, too—that would definitely drive the stress away!

3. Work the lungs out. In order to strengthen the lungs, you have to work them out, too. You could do this by doing deep-breathing exercises. Visualize how you'd inhale all the nutrients you need, as well as how you'd exhale toxins away. These will certainly help.

4. **Go to the sauna!** You could sweat it out at the sauna—which will easily rid your body of toxins, or brush the skin with sugar or salt. It would also be best if you could switch to all-organic beauty products. You do not need any artificial elements in your skin!

Chapter 8: It Doesn't End With Tea

Of course, the diet just doesn't end with all these different kinds of teas. You also have to keep in mind that you have to aid tea with the right kinds of food. In the last chapter of this book, you'll find a simple, easy to follow 3 week meal plan that you can use while drinking tea at designated times that have earlier been discussed, plus here are some tips that you also should keep in mind about the diet!

1. **Chew gassy vegetables and beans slowly.** Potatoes, sweet potatoes, yams, cauliflower, broccoli, and other cruciferous vegetables could make you gassy—so take your time in chewing them. By eating beans regularly, your body gets immune to the gassy feeling, just make sure that you add small amounts only.

2. **Chew your food slowly.** You know, most fast eaters end up with bloated bellies because they don't take time to chew their food. The thing with not chewing food slowly is that you end up sucking too much air which could then lead to bloating. So, just take your time. Remember, eating isn't a race—make sure that you enjoy your food, and that you eat properly.

3. **Don't drink carbonated drinks too much.** Carbonated drinks (even low-cal/diet ones) just trap gas inside your body, so if you're not a big

157

fan of water, you can spruce it up a bit by adding lime, lemon, or orange—to turn it into flavored water. Peppermint tea could also help, as well.

6. **Eat 5 to 6 small meals instead of 2 to 3 big meals.** Doing so would prevent you from feeling bloated, and would make it easy for your body to digest and metabolize what you have eaten. Plus, when you eat small meals, you get to prevent yourself from feeling hungry over and over again.

4. **Limit sodium intake.** Sodium is abundant in processed foods (i.e. junk foods, chips, soda, etc.) so it's important to minimize your intake of those. Another good tip is to make sure that you read food labels properly. Choose those that say "low-sodium" or "sodium-free". It's important to make sure that you do not take more than 500mg of sodium in a day.

5. **Look for sugar-free foods.** Bloating is also caused by taking too much alcohol and sugar-laden foods, so make sure that you don't take more than 2 to 3 servings of sugary foods per day.

2. **Stay away from chewing gum.** Chewing gum also makes you suck in more air than necessary. Sometimes, it's hard to stay away from chewing gum, though, because it's a habit of many, but what you can do is just choose other healthy foods, when you're in need of a good snack. Try low-fat popcorn, fruits, and vegetables instead.

8. **Try probiotics.** Probiotics are simply good bacteria that keep the immune system healthy, and prevent bloating by regulating digestive process. They also regulate the amount of good bacteria in the body, as well.

9. **Hydrate yourself.** At times when emotional hunger arises, do yourself a favor, and keep yourself hydrated. This way, toxins would be flushed away, and digestive processes would be regulated. You can also try working on a project, or going out just so you could distract yourself from eating more than you should.

Chapter 8: Sample Meal Plan

Finally, here is an easy to follow, 3-week meal plan that you can use to aid those teas in helping you lose weight and drive toxins away for good!

(Breakfast, Lunch, Snack, Dinner, Dessert)

Week 1

Day 1:

Jicama Apple Cinnamon Porridge

Classic Chicken Soup

Apple Chips

Quinoa Salad and Roasted Vegetables

Strawberry Date Cake

Day 2:

Peach Mango Shake

Vegetable and Bean Salad

Avocado Sandwich

Avocado and Chilled Carrot Soup with Sunflower Seed Pate

Apples in Maple Syrup

Day 3:

Kale and Spinach Shake

Fish Tacos

Oat and Strawberry Mix

Cucumber and Fennel Salad

Artichoke Tart

Day 4:

Chia Blueberry Shake

Cauliflower Rataouille

Carrot Sticks with Hummus

Slow Simmered Chicken with cherries, onions, mushrooms, and chard

Cherry Compote

Day 5:

Mango Banana Blueberry Smoothie

Salmon Fillets with Asparagus

Cauliflower roasted in curry

Vegetarian Nori Rolls with Nut Rice

Almond Meringues

Day 6:

Chili Apple Smoothie

Lamb Koftas with Tomatoes and Onions

Strawberry and Rhubarb Risotto

Kelp and Winter Squash Stew

Mango Pudding

Day 7:

Sweet Protein Shake

Radish and Arugula Crostini

Carrot Sticks with Peanut Butter

Winter Beet Soup

Basil Ice Cream

Week 2

Day 1:

Fruit and Mint Salad

Brussels Sprouts and Red Onion Salad with Apples

Kale Chips

Curried Red Lentil Vegetable Stew

Homemade Coconut Ice Cream

Day 2:

Dandelion Shake

Stir-Fried Chicken with Angelino Plums, Red Cabbage, and Water Chestnuts

Fermented Apple and Red Cabbage

Pan-Roasted Salmon

Banana Gelato

Day 3:

Asparagus and Chicken Crepes

Carrot and Black Bean Soup

Portobello Burgers with Goat Cheese

Sardines, Carrots, and Avocado with Mixed Greens

Banana and Berry Bowl

Day 4:

Grape and Banana Smoothie

Mushroom Steak with Wintergreen Salad

Sweet Potato Chips

Thai Vegetable Salad Wraps served with Almond Sauce

Watermelon Pudding

Day 5:

Chia and Blackberry Power Bars

Ginger and Vegetable Curry

Nacho Turkey Bake

Chicken Salad with Lavender Vinaigrette

Pineapple Upside Down Cake

Day 6:

Cilantro Shake

Celery Root Bisque and Wilted Winter Greens

Strawberry Gummies

Vegetable Lasagna with Cashew Cheese

Pecan-Toffee Pudding

Day 7:

Peach Blueberry Kale Smoothie

Tuna Salad Lettuce Wraps

Quinoa and Broccoli Bites

Crabless Cakes

Pumpkin Spiced Doughnuts

Week 3

Day 1:

Blueberry and Almond Shake

Pulled Chicken with Cabbage Slaw

Onion and Flaxseed Crackers

Leek and Asparagus Bisque

Carrot Cake Cookies

Day 2:

Roasted Cabbage Wedges

Purple Cabbage and Avocado Salad

Chickpeas roasted in maple

Sweet Potato, Kale, and Lentil Slaw

Oat and Strawberry Squares

Day 3:

Cucumber and Ginger Juice

Sunflower Seed and Cauliflower Salad

Kale and Spicy Rice Bowl

Fruit Kebabs

Melon and Mango Fruit Bowl

Day 4:

Charred Tomatoes on Garlic Toast

Squash and Arugula Salad

Vegan Pesto

Halibut and Lime Salad

Apricot Sorbet

Day 5:

Mango Ginger Shake

Olive and Fennel Salad

Carrot Sticks with Pea-Mint Dip

Chipotle and Black Bean Bisque

Orange and Pineapple Salad with Toasted Coconut

Day 6:

Acorn with Chili-Lime Vinaigrette

Apple, Lamb, and Onion Skewers

Brown Rice Nachos

Stuffed Eggplant with Tahini Sauce

Grapefruit Granita

Day 7:

Cashew Dandelion Shake

Salmon Quesadillas with Avocado-Peach Sauce

Roasted Beets

Chickpea Enchiladas

Raspberry Ice Pops

Chapter 9: Why You Likely Need A Tea Cleanse

To better understand why you may need to consider a detoxifying tea cleanse, it is important to understand the Standard American Diet and how it is killing you.

As far as daily nutrition routines go, the diet most American's consists on isn't just unhealthy, it is one of the least healthy in the entire world. As such, the term Standard American Diet is academic shorthand for the type of diet which includes a high amount of saturated fats, excessive animal fats and too much processed foods.

In addition, it contains only small amount of vegetables, fruits, fiber and complex carbohydrates. Perhaps unsurprisingly, this type of diet is known to cause an increase in the risk of cancer, heart disease and stroke. What's more surprising is that as the Standard American Diet gains hold in a new area, these increased rates of disease and risk of disease begin showing up in as little as 5 years.

Is it any wonder we all have a heavy toxic load inside of us just waiting for a good detoxification?

It is perhaps too ironic that scientists around the world have spent countless hours researching a cure for cancer when a quick and easy way to reduce its chances of appearing have been staring them in the face every day as they head out to lunch.

Over the past four decades the Standard American Diet has come to include more than 25 percent more calories than it used to. A recent study found that almost three-fourths of all meals purchased while "eating out" came from fast-food establishments and that half of those included a hamburger and more than 30 percent included a drink that is either loaded with sugar in the form of high fructose corn syrup or an alternative that is statistically likely to increase the risk of health problems.

America can now be considered a fast food culture and Americans seem blissfully unware of the fact that the quality of the fats, proteins and carbohydrates they put into their bodies is just as important as the quantity, if not even more so.

Nutritionists theorize that for each and every percent of saturated fat removed from your diet and replaced with positive fats found in things like fish, nuts or leafy greens you can decrease your odds of contracting a coronary heart disease by upwards of 5 percent.

The other major issue with the Standard American Diet is the way in which it forces processed foods upon the masses at an alarming rate. A food can be considered processed if any part of that food has been treated with any chemicals, regardless of their purpose.

Items that are made from refined products are also considered processed. Only when all of the ingredients in an item are completely natural can the food be considered real instead of processed.

Processed foods tend to have between three and four times as much sugar as their unprocessed doppelgangers. This added sugar adds nothing of value to the food, it only increases its calories and the number of toxins it holds. When consumed in too large of quantiles it is known to increase the amount of harmful cholesterol found in the blood, fatty buildup on the liver and type 2 diabetes.

The other main warning sign of processed foods is the amount of refined carbohydrates they contain. These carbohydrates contain significantly less nutritional value than complex carbohydrates and as a result provide significantly less energy when used to fuel the body.

The worst part of all is that modern food companies are aware of just what they are doing to people and they are only interested in packing in more sugar and fat in hopes of tricking more people in becoming addicted to their products.

This works because back when humans were still hunter/gatherers, find foods that were high in sugar or fat was a good way of gauging if it was high in essential vitamins and nutrients as well. This is no longer the case however, and in fact, the opposite is true.

This is why it is possible to eat an entire bag of fast food and still feel hungry afterwards. During your detox you may feel elements of withdrawal as your body works its way off of processed food, this is because modern processed foods are nearly as addictive as cigarettes and twice as hard to quit for good.

When looking for foods to avoid, consider all nonorganic meats and vegetables as more trouble than they are worth. The variety of chemicals and pesticides used on these products will fill the body full of toxins at a rate that practically negates all of the nutritional benefits they might have once contained.

Likewise, refined flour is the surest sign a product is lousy with refined carbohydrates. These products are also more likely to be full of toxins, including the gluten itself. If you plan on getting the most out of a tea cleanse, these should be some of the first things to go.

Chapter 10: Tea Cleanse Basics

Tea, be it green or black, can be related to health benefits which span nearly the entire body. For starters it helps to facility weight loss and decrease your risk of heart disease and stroke while at the same time improving mental performance, enhancing mood and lowering blood pressure.

However, when it comes to long-term detoxification and weight loss, tea is only one part of the puzzle. You need to ensure that you are eating and exercising in such a way that the tea can do its job properly.

With that being said, both types of tea are full of antioxidants which is what makes them so effective when it comes to enhancing the body's natural detoxification process. In fact, the natural boosting effects of tea means that you can get just as much benefit from detoxification teas you make at home (as discussed in chapter 4) as you can from teas sold online which can cost up to $10 per bag.

Again, it is important to note that a tea cleanse can only do so much on its own, you need to eat healthy and exercise regularly to see any type of real results.

Another thing to remember when it comes to a tea cleanse is that the diuretic effect of the tea coupled with its caffeine content will mean that a fair portion of the weight you lose will be water weight. While you will still look better for a time after the cleanse it is important to remember that, strictly speaking, you won't be just losing fat.

Likewise, the laxative effect of the tea will help expunge stored waste from your intestines which will make your stomach seem flatter but the losses aren't from body fat so their overall effect is more for confidence boosting than productive weight loss. What this means is that unless you change your habits as well, any effect you notice from the detox tea will most likely be temporary.

When you are considering various types of teas in hopes of removing toxins from your body, it is important to carefully consider all of the ingredients to ensure you are not accidentally doing yourself more harm than good.

Many teas include a variety of herbs in hopes of improve metabolism while at the same time decreasing appetite. Many of these herbs can have other side effects including Senna, a common natural laxative which when taken for prolonged periods of time can lead to dehydration, electrolyte imbalance, diarrhea and even vomiting.

Another common detoxification ingredient to be wary of is guarana which can cause ringing in the ears, increased rate of breathing, stomach irritation, headache, nausea or anxiety, especially if you are already sensitive to caffeine. When mixed with tea's natural caffeine guarana, can also make it more difficult for you to sleep, especially during a prolonged cleanse.

This is an important issue to pay attention to because your body enjoys a routine. If you are on a regular sleep cycle before you cleanse and then are suddenly sleeping at different hours or for different amounts of time your body may get confused and try and hold on to everything it has right now until it figures out what is going on. What this means for your cleanse is that it may be a bust if you vary to radically from your normal habits.

Regardless of what type of tea you choose, the most effective times to consume it are first thing in the morning and before your evening meal to ensure the body is as empty, and thus primed for the oxidation process, as possible.

Depending on how sensitive you are to caffeine, you can probably handle several more cups than just 2. An average number of cups to consume during a cleanse should be between 5 and 7 per day.

If you are interested in the idea of cleansing but are not quite sure if it is for you, here are a few questions to help you make up your mind.

Do you have some weight that just won't leave?

If no matter what you do, you just can't get rid of that those last few pounds then it might be you are coming at the problem the wrong way.

Many toxins latch on to the bodies fat and then set up shop, making it impossible to lose that weight in a traditional manner. If you have been battling the same bit of fat for as long as you can remember, a tea cleanse can help sort you out.

Are you more exhausted than you should be at the end of the day?

If you feel as though you are getting enough sleep and yet you still feel tired in the morning or if you feel more exhausted at the end of the day than you should the cause could be toxins in the body.

Carrying around a high amount of toxins means your body needs to work harder for the same results, which ultimately leads to exhaustion. The stress from an excessive toxic load can put too much pressure on your adrenal gland leaving you with the worn out feeling you have come to know and loathe. If this sounds like you then a tea cleanse can ease your body's toxic load.

Do you find yourself unable to get to sleep at night?

When your body is dealing with a high amount of toxins for a prolonged period of time it can lead to a fluctuation in your cortisol levels when in turn will make it difficult to sleep properly. As such, you may find yourself with way too much energy at all hours of the night.

If you find yourself unable to sleep, a tea cleanse may be just what you need.

Do you have a hard time concentrating or have too many headaches?

If you are suffering for a high level of toxins in your body, then there is a good chance some of those including aspartame and MSG found in some foods may be affecting your brain in a negative way.

If you find it difficult to concentrate throughout the day or if you have several unexplained headaches, then a tea cleanse may be just what you need.

Do you find yourself changing moods rapidly?

If you are carrying a heavy toxic load, then the reason for your rapid mood swings may be a hormonal imbalance caused by toxins that react like estrogen in the body. In addition to a tea cleanse, cutting down on the amount of plastics that touch your food will also help.

Has your body odor gotten worse?

If you find that your breath or bowel movements are carrying a more particular aroma than normal, this can be a sign that your body is suffering under a heavy toxic load. As a result, your liver and colon are having difficulty meeting the demand which accounts for the unexpected issues.

In addition to a tea detox milk thistle can help them both process toxins more effectively.

Are your muscles inexplicably sore?

Many toxins activate the pain receptors in various parts of the body and carrying a heavy toxic load can make many of these receptors light up at once. If you find yourself with lots of new knots in your muscles or find you are having muscle spasms, then it might be time to consider a tea detox.

Are you more sensitive to different smells than you have been before?

An increased sensitivity to smell is a sign that your liver is having a hard time removing all of the toxins from your system. If you find this is the case, consider switching to a more organic diet before trying out a tea cleanse.

Chapter 11: Getting Started

The idea of a period of time dedicated exclusively to detoxifying the body as effectively as possible is certainly effective, but it is certainly not the only way to put tea's antioxidant effects to work for you.

Regardless of your goals when it comes to drinking more tea, the first is to decide if you prefer green tea or black tea. Both are made from the camellia Sinesis plant though the different methods by which each is processed lead to substantially different results.

Black Tea

Unlike green tea, black tea leaves are withered, rolled and heated before ultimately being fermented prior to use. Black tea offers up a variety of benefits which make it a great choice to add into your daily diet.

It is important to drink black tea straight in order to see the most positive results.

- Black tea has been shown to reduce the amount of plaque that forms on the teeth by mitigating the growth of the bacteria which causes it.
- The unique antioxidants found in black tea have been shown to help prevent the damage smoking does to the DNA.

- Woman who make it a habit of drinking black tea have a statistically lower chance of developing ovarian cancer.
- Drinking as few as two cups of black tea per day can reduce your risk of diabetes by nearly 75 percent.
- Black tea moderates' cortisol production which makes it better at reducing stress and promoting healthy sleep.
- The alkylamine in black tea boosts the immune system and helps to combat viruses.

Green Tea

Green tea is considered the healthier of the teas because the fermentation process that black tea is subjected to mitigates many of its health benefits.

Green tea is a better choice for a dedicated detoxification process because it contains more oxidizing and antioxidant elements.

- As discussed in detail in chapter 5, green tea is known to improve the metabolism and maximize weight loss.
- Green tea has been shown to moderate glucose levels which means it can help mitigate the effect of type 2 diabetes.
- Green tea has been show to improve the lining of blood vessels which can help prevent against clots and maintain a steady blood pressure. Taken together they help to decrease the risk of heart attacks.

- Green tea has been shown to kill cancer cells and is especially effective when mitigating esophageal cancer.
- Green tea has been show to decrease the amount of bad cholesterol in the blood.
- Studies on mice show that green tea can prevent the deterioration of brain cells four in both Parkinson's and Alzheimer's disease.
- Green tea has been shown to decrease feelings of depression.
- Green tea has been shown to reduce wrinkles and other signs of aging. It also works as a topical cream to reduce damage caused by extreme exposure to the sun.

Get ready to detox

Any good detoxification process should consist of a morning tea which is all about getting you ready to start your day and an evening tea which in turn is all about getting your body to expel as many toxins as possible.

The morning tea should also include plenty of electrolytes and vitamins to replace those lost during the cleanse. When deciding on a morning tea focus on those which contain lots of vitamin and antioxidants, teas with barley grass, ginseng, acai berry or spirulina are all valid choices.

When it comes to choosing an evening tea it is important to choose one that contains plenty of diuretics to ensure you get rid of as many of the toxins and other harmful junk hiding in your body as possible. The most important thing to look for in an evening tea is Senna leaf.

Remember, it is important to consume Senna in moderation as too much can quickly become harmful to the body. Additional beneficial ingredients to look for when it comes to an evening tea is licorice root lemon grass, nettle leaves, dandelion greens and orange peel which has been dried.

All of these chose will add a great flavor to the tea while at the same time strengthening its effects.

Chapter 12: Detox Tea Recipes

Basic Detox Tea

This tea is especially great at getting rid of that bloated feeling. It is also useful for improving metabolism, decreasing blood pressure and maintain a steady blood sugar level. It is easy to make and almost everyone should already have all of the ingredients required.

What's in it

- Lemon to taste
- Honey (1 teaspoon)
- Hot Water
- Apple Cider Vinegar (1 tablespoon)

Ginger Detox Tea

This recipe gets the job done with the addition of ginger and cayenne, a detox tea with a kick.

What's in it

- Hot Water (12 ounces)
- Ginger Root (2 ounces peeled)
- Cinnamon (1 stick)
- Cloves (2)
- Cayenne Extract (2 drops)
- Honey (1 teaspoon)
- Lemon Juice (to taste)

Iced Detox Tea

This recipe is completely paleo diet friendly in addition to being a great way to start or end a day of detoxing. Allow all of the ingredients to steep until the water has cooled.

This recipe makes enough to that you have plenty of water on hand to get your daily recommended dose for a total of 9 servings.

What's in it

- Boiling Water (9 cups)
- Lemon (2 juiced)
- Ginger (5 coins)
- Honey (3 tablespoons)
- Basil leaves (.75 cups)

Mint Detox Tea

This tea is all about options, it is easy to vary its potency and it is as tasty warm as it is cooled. This recipe makes about 2 cups of tea with 3 minutes of preparation and 5 minutes of cooking. The remainder of the dry blend will make about 4 pots of tea total.

What's in it

- Lemon (3 thin slices)
- Mint Leaves (16)
- Ginger (3 coins)
- Black Peppercorns (2 teaspoons)
- Cumin Seeds (1.5 teaspoons)
- Fennel Seeds (4 teaspoons)
- Coriander Seeds (4 teaspoons)

How's it made

- Mix the seeds and the peppercorn together and set to one side.
- Start 2 cups of water simmering and while it heats break up the mint and ginger.
- Add the mint/ginger and dry mixture to water to taste.
- Simmer for 5 minutes
- Steep for 3 minutes
- Add lemon to taste

Detox Smoothie

With a green tea base, this smoothie is a delicious and effective way to mix up your tea detox in a meaningful (and tasty way).

This recipe makes 2 smoothies and takes about five minutes to prepare. Blend all of the ingredients together in a blender.

What's in it

- Ice (.5 cups)
- Vanilla Extract (.5 teaspoon)
- Honey (1 tablespoon)
- Banana (1 peeled)
- Raspberries (.5 pints)
- Yogurt (.3 cups)
- Green Tea (1 cup chilled)

Chapter 13: Green Tea Challenge

While celebrities are often known to tout the benefits of a green tea challenge, whereby you drink between 5 and 10 cups of green tea per day for 10 days as a weight loss method, it is important to remember that green tea is only part of the equation.

Remember to maintain a healthy diet during the challenge and also to exercise regularly. In order to ensure you are losing weight in a way which will not damage your body in the long term it is crucial to never consume less than 1200 calories per day, especially while you are exercising.

Remember, in order to lose a pound of weight you need to burn 3,500 calories, it is up to you how you choose to do so.

Diet Plan

While committing to drinking green tea is helpful, if you do not make an effort to change your diet during this period as well, you will only be replacing the toxins you have work so hard to remove.

As such it is important to alter your diet so it is largely comprised of fresh fruits and vegetables. Lean protein is also a good choice and this can include either fish or turkey, chicken, lamb or pork.

If you are looking for a healthy snack, unsalted nuts including pine nuts, almonds, pistachios, walnuts and peanuts are all good options. Fill out your diet by including things like brown rice, oats tofu and seeds.

Likewise, it is important to avoid foods which are high in fat including eggs, milk, cream, margarine, butter and cheese. It is important to avoid gluten during your cleanse which means all forms of bread should be avoided as much as possible.

Sugar and coffee should both be avoided as should soda, salt, mayonnaise, pickles and squash.

Get serious

A 10-day tea challenge is enough time to allow your body to begin to adjust to a healthier lifestyle but a 30-day challenge is enough to allow you to build new habits that could potentially last a lifetime.

Regardless, it is important to prepare before you start to ensure you have plenty of tea and healthy food options to get you through the first leg of your challenge.

The easiest way to eat something you'll regret is to find yourself suddenly out of healthy options and without the time to go shopping. If you do eat something you regret it is important to brush it off and keep at it, the only time you should feel bad about a little slipup is if you use it as an excuse to quit the challenge completely.

It is important to ensure that your bowel movements remain regular and that you stick to the routine or a revitalizing tea in the morning and a cleansing tea at night. The detoxification process should be processing out more toxins then normal and as such it is normal for your bowel movements to increase substantially.

Be sure to keep this fact in mind and increase your nutrient intake and water consumption accordingly. While on a challenge it is important to try and drink a gallon of water every day. At the start of the challenge your body might become constipated in response to the change in diet; if this happens, consider a natural laxative but use it sparingly, it shouldn't take much to get your body primed for action.

Consider the type of exercise that is right for you, if you are attempting a low calorie diet, ensure you do not exercise so much that you end up burning muscle instead of fat.

A good place to start is with between 2 and 3 hours of cardio training per week combined with at least 3 days of strength training at around a moderate level of exertion. Exercising at your peak requires a large number of calories per day, and if you plan on putting on a lot of muscle it is important to increase your protein intake accordingly.

If you are exercising daily, it is important to consume at least 50 grams of protein per day to ensure your muscles get all of the fuel they need.

Before you begin any type of challenge it is important to assess how its methods align with your goals. It is important to always discuss your plans with a healthcare professional to ensure you get the most out of any challenge.

Women who are pregnant or nursing and those with a history of heart disease, liver disease or kidney problems should not consider a tea challenge regardless of the number of days it is meant to last as it can easily deprive the body of essential vitamins and nutrients.

Some medications can present side-effects when exposed to the high amount of caffeine found in green tea always know what you are taking before starting any challenge.

Conclusion

Thank you again for downloading this book!

I hope this book was able to help you to understand the tea cleanse diet, see what it can do for you, and appreciate the many amazing benefits of tea for your health!

The next step is to make sure that aside from reading this book, you'd also try the mentioned teas by yourself—and that you'd adhere to the 3-week meal plan. That way, you'd definitely lose weight in just 3 weeks!

Thank you and good luck with your cleanse !

www.ingramcontent.com/pod-product-compliance
Lightning Source LLC
Chambersburg PA
CBHW062137020426
42335CB00013B/1235